Atrial Fibrillation - Diagnosis and Management in the 21st Century

Edited by Özgür Karcıoğlu and Funda Karbek Akarca

Published in London, United Kingdom

Atrial Fibrillation - Diagnosis and Management in the 21st Century
http://dx.doi.org/10.5772/intechopen.100927
Edited by Özgür Karcıoğlu and Funda Karbek Akarca

Contributors
Serkan Asil, Edidiong Orok, Funmilayo Adeniyi, Oluwole Akawa, Manuel Lorenzo López Reboiro, Raul Franco Gutierrez, Laura Ramos Rua, Maria del Carmen Basalo Carbajales, Laura Rodrigo Lara, Candela Fraga González, Celia Sobrado Moreiras, Jose Manuel Cerqueiro González, Jose López Castro, Kohei Sawasaki, Dian Andina Munawar, Anggia Chairuddin Lubis, Muhammad Munawar, Jonathan Tardos, Amit H. Patel, Amanda Chajkowski, Nawal Aamir, Dhaval Desai, Chawannuch Ruaengsri, Suchart Chaiyaroj, Julio Garcia, Mankarman Ghuman, Hansuk Kim, Hana Sheitt, Nayanjyoti Kaushik, James Arter Chapman, Andrew Gillaspie, Stephen Ackerman, Peter Gallagher, Deobrat Mallick, Steven J. Bailin, Andrea Rossi, Marcello Piacenti, Procolo Marchese, Özgür Karcıoğlu

First published in London, United Kingdom, 2022 by IntechOpen
IntechOpen is the global imprint of INTECHOPEN LIMITED, registered in England and Wales, registration number: 11086078, 5 Princes Gate Court, London, SW7 2QJ, United Kingdom

British Library Cataloguing-in-Publication Data
A catalogue record for this book is available from the British Library

Additional hard and PDF copies can be obtained from orders@intechopen.com

Atrial Fibrillation - Diagnosis and Management in the 21st Century
Edited by Özgür Karcıoğlu and Funda Karbek Akarca
p. cm.
Print ISBN 978-1-80356-122-6
Online ISBN 978-1-80356-123-3
eBook (PDF) ISBN 978-1-80356-124-0

For EU product safety concerns:
IN TECH d.o.o., Prolaz Marije Krucifikse Kozulić 3, 51000 Rijeka, Croatia,
info@intechopen.com or visit our website at intechopen.com.

Meet the editors

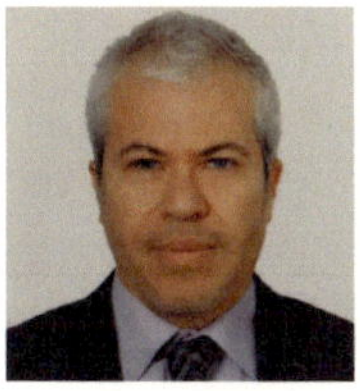

Özgür Karcıoğlu graduated from the residency program at the Department of Emergency Medicine, Dokuz Eylul University Medical School, Turkey, in 1998. He obtained an International Emergency Medicine Fellowship at Penn State University in 2005. He is currently chair of the Department of Emergency Medicine, Taksim Education and Research Hospital, Turkey. He has served as a founder and board member of the Emergency Medical Association of Turkey since 1995. His research interests include resuscitation, advanced life support, pain management, airway emergencies, disaster medicine, trauma and toxicology, and diagnosis and management of COVID-19. He has published more than 160 articles in scientific journals, and his h-index is 24 in the year 2022. In addition to four edited volumes with IntechOpen, he has authored three books, *Diagnosis and Treatment of COVID-19, Cardiac Care in Medical Practice and Acute Abdominal Pain,* published by Bentham Science Publishers.

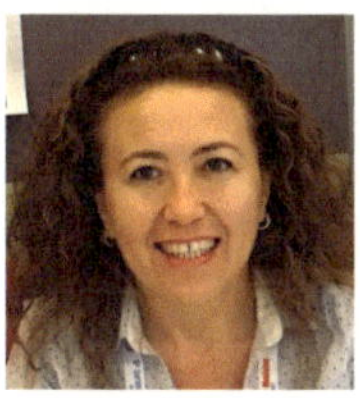

Funda Karbek Akarca graduated from the Department of Emergency Medicine, Dokuz Eylul University, in 2005. She worked as an emergency physician at the İzmir Atatürk Training and Research Hospital from 2006 to 2010. She has been a faculty member in the Department of Emergency Medicine at Ege University since 2010. She was the founding member of the ultrasonography working group of the Emergency Medical Association of Turkey, serving as its chairman for two terms. She also works as an instructor in disaster medicine and critical care working groups. She has published 35 articles and ten book chapters and edited three books.

Contents

Preface

Cardiovascular disease is among the most prominent health issues worldwide and remains the leading cause of death in the developed world. It has also become an increasing threat in developing countries in recent decades. It is of vital importance to increase awareness of the risk factors for this disease, and to alleviate probable challenges and complications while improving outcomes.

The medical community has witnessed major advances in cardiac biomarkers, electrocardiographic monitoring, ultrasonography/echocardiography and other bedside diagnostic tools, defibrillation, and other strategies to curb the mortality resulting from cardiac diseases in general as well as from acute and chronic atrial fibrillation (AF). Important short- and long-term complications can ensue in a patient with AF, whether or not a diagnosis has been established. Timely management of this supraventricular arrhythmia will alleviate complications attributed to AF, such as thromboembolic disease, heart failure, and others. This book aims to demonstrate advances in the diagnosis of AF and other supraventricular arrhythmias, and to delineate pathways to their optimal management. Special procedures to prevent thromboembolic complications are also covered.

The book is divided into two sections, representing diagnostic and therapeutic aspects of these diseases and special procedures pursued within the scope of the project. The chapters in **Section 1, "Principles of Diagnosis and Management of Atrial Fibrillation"**, examine principles of recognition and treatment of supraventricular arrhythmias both in general medical practice and in emergency medicine. The pros and cons of rhythm control strategies and prevention of thromboembolism via dual antiplatelet therapy are described.

Section 2, "Special Procedures in the Treatment of Atrial Fibrillation", covers advanced invasive interventions, including cryoablation, vein of Marshall alcoholization, and surgical ablation, aimed at a permanent solution for supraventricular arrhythmias. Left atrial appendage (LAA) occlusion or closure is a procedure that blocks the LAA opening to prevent thromboembolism in selected susceptible patients.

The book not only focuses on atrial arrhythmias but also provides invaluable opinions and advice on the management of cardiac emergencies for both the general readership and specialists. The medical community is sure to find the contents useful both in acute settings and in the interventional laboratory.

Özgür Karcıoğlu
Department of Emergency Medicine,
University of Health Sciences,
Taksim Training and Research Hospital,
Beyoglu, Istanbul, Turkey

Funda Karbek Akarca
Associate Professor,
School of Medicine,
Emergency Department,
Ege University,
Bornova, Izmir, Turkey

Section 1

Principles of Diagnosis and Management of Atrial Fibrillation

Chapter 1

Recognition and Management of Supraventricular Arrhythmias and Atrial Fibrillation in the Acute Setting

Özgür Karcıoğlu

Abstract

Supraventricular tachycardia (SVT) is a type of tachyarrhythmia with a narrow QRS complex and regular rhythm. These patients are often symptomatic and present to the emergency department (ED) due to acute attacks called paroxysmal SVT. Attacks of SVT start suddenly with the reentry mechanism in most patients. Anginal chest pain and dyspnea occur in patients due to tachycardia. Vagal manoeuvers and adenosine is the treatments of choice for termination of SVT. In multifocal atrial tachycardia (MAT), at least three different P wave morphologies are observed in the ECG, along with variable PP, PR and RR intervals. Treatment is to correct the underlying disease. Patients with atrial flutter (AFl) tend to come to the ED with unstable findings. Atrial fibrillation (AF) is the term used to define the inactive 'worm bag-like' oscillations of the atria, with an absence of true atrium contraction. Ruling out atrial or ventricular thrombi with echocardiography is important to avoid embolization. Priority should be given to hemodynamic stability and the determination of factors triggering the underlying disease. IV beta-blocker and diltiazem can be used for rate control in AF with rapid ventricular response.

Keywords: arrhythmia, supraventricular tachycardia, atrial fibrillation, atrial flutter, narrow QRS complex, palpitations, vagal manoeuvers, adenosine

1. Introduction

Supraventricular tachycardias (SVT) are a type of arrhythmia defined with a narrow QRS complex (<120 msec) and regular tachycardia [>100 beats per minute (bpm)]. Erroneous impulse formation and abnormalities in the conduction pathways (known as reentry mechanism) are blamed for their pathophysiology. Patients may be admitted with a wide range of symptoms, from minor palpitations to severe symptoms such as hypotension and altered mental status. Complaints can last from a few minutes to hours. They often present to the emergency department (ED) due to acute episodes known as paroxysmal SVT (PSVT).

The incidence of SVT is approximately 1–3 cases per 1000 persons and its prevalence increases with age [1]. Atrioventricular (AV) Nodal Reentrant Tachycardia (AVNRT) is most common in middle age and older, while SVT with accessory conduction is more common in younger patients. PSVT can also be triggered by coronary artery disease, myocardial infarction (MI), mitral valve regurgitation (MVR), rheumatic heart disease, pericarditis, chronic obstructive pulmonary disease (COPD) and intoxications via alcohol/caffeine/energy drink.

2. Diagnostic characteristics

Ectopic SVT usually originates in the atrium and the atrial velocity is 100–250 bpm (mostly recorded to be between 140 and 200 bpm). Regular P waves may be misdiagnosed as atrial flutter or 2:1 AV block, sinus rhythm. Sixty-percent of the patients have reentry with AV node, and 20% have reentry via bypass pathways. In SVT, QRS complex is narrow (<0.12 seconds), or wide in conjunction with a previously known branch/fascicular block or rate-dependent aberrant conduction.

Reentrant SVT usually starts when the AV node encounters an ectopic atrial impulse while the AV node is in the partial refractory period. From here, the impulse proceeds with two different functional parallel arms (**Figure 1**). The node is below the ventricular ending and above the atrium. In the case of AV nodal reentry, QRS complexes usually hide the P waves and are not visible. These have a 1:1 message and QRS complexes are normal (**Table 1**).

Ectopic SVT can be seen in patients with acute MI, chronic lung disease, pneumonia, alcohol or digoxin intoxication (often associated with AV block). Atrial tachycardia with block is also frequently (75%) associated with digoxin toxicity. Reentrant SVT is mostly associated with normal heart or rheumatic heart disease, acute pericarditis, MI, and MVR.

2.1 Clinical course and findings

Tachycardia is usually the only finding in those with normal hemodynamic reserve. A previously 'normal' heart can tolerate a 'typical' SVT rate of 160–200 bpm in a given timeframe. However, cardiac output is generally decreased and may lead to signs of heart failure (HF) in the intact myocardium in those with high heart rates. Coronary artery disease, chest pain and dyspnea occur in patients due to tachycardia. Heart failure and pulmonary edema may occur with decreased left ventricular function. In the presence of right heart failure, tachypnea, hypotension, third heart sound (S3), jugular venous distension (JVD), peripheral edema and hepatomegaly may be observed.

Although serious signs such as loss of consciousness and syncope increase the risk, SVT is generally not a severe or life-threatening condition. The most common complaints encountered in symptomatic patients presenting with PSVT are as follows: palpitation (96%), dizziness/lightheadedness (75%), dyspnea (47%) and chest pain (35%). Patients with a heart rate above 170 bpm may experience dizziness and syncope.

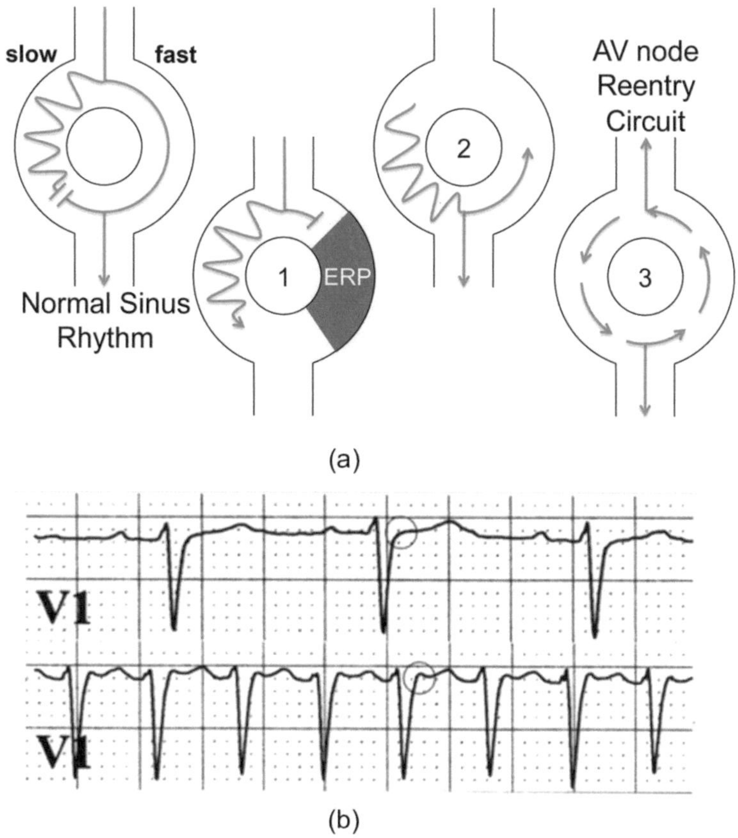

Figure 1.
(a) Re-entry mechanism in AVNRT. Among the subtypes, the most common type is slow-fast re-entrant type AVNRT. (b) ECG findings of this type of SVT:P waves are often hidden in QRS complexes, a false R′ wave (pseudo-R) may be seen in V1 and/or V2 and false S waves (pseudo-S) may be seen in II, III, aVF.

2.2 Evaluation and history

Since the hypotensive event and episode of hypoxia may have triggered the arrhythmia, the history should be extended in terms of diseases such as gastrointestinal bleeding, ruptured ectopic pregnancy, carbon monoxide poisoning and pneumonia, especially in cases presenting with the first attack. Drugs such as nitrate or diuretic, phosphodiesterase inhibitors (PDEI)-5 (sildenafil), alpha-blocker that may cause new onset hypotension should also be questioned in history.

2.3 Laboratory

Further examination of the patients who are stable at admission and have been converted to NSR immediately is unnecessary in the emergency setting. Cardiac enzymes should be evaluated in patients with risk factors for MI, those presenting with chest pain, unstable patients and patients with HF, hypotension, and pulmonary edema. A complete blood count (CBC) is useful in showing anaemia

Tachycardias	A/AV	ECG findings
Sinus tachycardia	A	Heart rate > 100/min Sinus rhythm (P waves) Regular PR intervals
Inappropriate sinus tachycardia (IST)	A	Similar to sinus tachycardia Sinus rhythm (P waves)
Sinus nodal reentrant tachycardia	A	Sudden start and end Sinus rhythm (P waves)
Atrial tachycardia	A	Heart rate 120–250/min P waves with different configurations Prolonged PR interval
Multifocal atrial tachycardia	A	Heart rate > 100–200/min Three different P wave morphologies
Atrial flutter	A	Atrial rate 200–300/min Sawtooth flutter waves AV conduction ratio 2:1 or 4:1
Atrial fibrillation	A	Irregular rhythm P waves are not visible
Atrioventricular nodal reentrant tachycardia	AV	Heart rate 150–200/min P wave inside or immediately after the QRS complex Short PR interval in typical AVNRT Long PR interval in atypical AVNRT
Atrioventricular reentrant tachycardia	AV	Heart rate 150–250/min Narrow QRS complexes in orthodromic conduction Wide QRS complexes in antidromic conduction P waves after the QRS complex

Table 1.
The differential diagnosis of narrow QRS tachycardia with ECG findings in patients presenting with PSVT. (A) Denotes atrial tachyarrhythmias and (AV) atrioventricular tachyarrhythmias.

that can cause ischemia or tachycardia. Thyroid function tests can be used to rule out hyperthyroidism. Serum digoxin levels should be checked in patients using the agent.

2.4 Subtypes of SVT

If the reentry circuit is within the atrial myocardium; atrial fibrillation, atrial flutter, and some types of atrial tachycardia may occur. In this situation, AV node suppressing agents slow down the tachyarrhythmia but do not convert it.

In some re-entry tachycardias, the reentry circuit is in the AV node. These arrhythmias, which are characterized by a sudden onset and end, are recognized with a resting heart rate of over 150 bpm.

- AV nodal reentry tachycardia (AVNRT) occurs when both arms of the reentry circuit are in the AV node; the typical finding is that P waves cannot be discerned in this form (**Figure 1B**).

- One arm of the reentry circuit is in the accessory pathway and the other is in the AV node, called 'AV reentry tachycardia' (AVRT).

- AVNRT and AVRT are both PSVT.

- If at least one branch of the circuit is in the AV node, AV node suppressing agents will have a chance to terminate the arrhythmia.

- Another group called automatic tachycardias are generated due to an excited automatic stimulus focus, including ectopic atrial tachycardia, MAT and junctional tachycardias. Termination of these will be more gradual and slower. These do not respond to electrical cardioversion (ECV), furthermore, these are arrhythmias for which ECV is contraindicated. These are treated with rate control with agents that slow down AV conduction.

2.5 Imaging

Triggering diseases and infections such as edema and pneumonia can be displayed on chest radiography. Point-of-care ultrasound (POCUS)/echocardiography may be useful in suspected structural heart disease.

3. Treatment

First choice should be vagal manoeuvers (VM) followed by adenosine for termination of stable PSVT. The most common practical applications for this purpose in the context of VM include carotid sinus massage (CSM) and Valsalva. Apart from these, there are also techniques such as cold-water immersion and massage on the eyeball, which used to be more common in the past (**Figure 2**).

The VM slows down the AV node and lengthens the refractory period within the node. It also has a negative inotropic effect on the ventricular myocardium. VM is also indicated for the examination of cardiac murmurs.

3.1 Valsalva manoeuver and simplified modified Valsalva (SMV)

Valsalva manoeuver is the most commonly used VM because it is easy and practical. In most guidelines, it is primarily recommended for regular tachycardia treatment with narrow QRS. It is more successful in AVRT than AVNRT. Valsalva should not be administered to patients whose hemodynamic stability is not attained, those with known aortic stenosis, recent MI, and those who have diseases in which an increase in venous pressures may be dangerous.

Different percentages (19–54%) are reported for clinical success rate. Although a Cochrane review recently announced that there is insufficient evidence to support or refute its effectiveness, it is widely used all over the world [2]. In a recent multicentric controlled study in China, SMV was found to be 43% successful and standard Valsalva 17% successful in terminating PSVT.

For standard Valsalva, the patient with stable narrow QRS and regular tachycardia sits in a comfortable position. After inspiration with normal tidal volume, it is asked to try to move the piston for 15 seconds by blowing into the injector with a 10- or 20-ml needle removed (trying to reach a pressure of 40 mmHg).

SMV is commenced in a semi-sitting position, after blowing for 15 seconds, the patient assumes a supine position and the legs are passively lifted concurrently. After

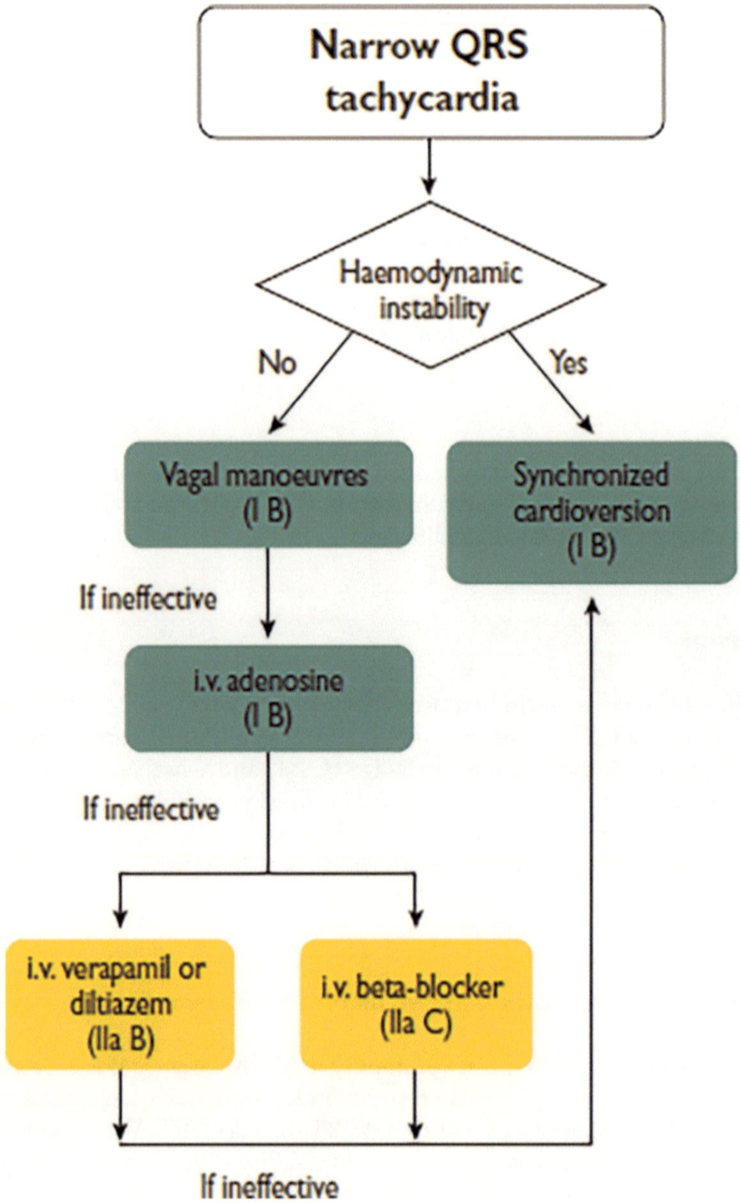

Figure 2.
Algorithm for emergency treatment of narrow-QRS tachycardia in the absence of previously established diagnosis.

waiting in this way for 15–30 seconds, the resting period starts, and the process is completed in around 1 minute.

CSM is applied under monitoring in the supine position, unilaterally with the neck facing the opposite side and in extension. The procedure can be performed with or without Valsalva manoeuver. At the carotid bulb where the carotid pulsation is taken, rubbing is performed with gentle pressure, without occluding the arterial flow. The process is completed in 5 seconds in a posteromedial direction, aiming toward the vertebral column. Double-sided procedure is absolutely contraindicated. It is not attempted in patients with a history of transient ischemic attack (TIA), stroke and a murmur in the carotid artery area.

CSM is applied to clarify the diagnosis, especially in syncope work up, in people who are thought to have a sensitive carotid sinus. Hypersensitive carotid sinus findings comprise persistent asystole or a drop in systolic blood pressure > 50 mmHg, lasting for at least 3 seconds just after CSM.

3.2 Drug therapy

Six-milligrams of adenosine is given via IV route in patients with PSVT who do not respond to the VM (Class I, LOE B). Then 20 ml of saline is flushed via the same vein. If sinus rhythm is not restored within 1–2 minutes, repeat 12 mg of the agent [3]. Continuous ECG monitoring is required to keep track of the rhythm.

In case of continuation of SVT or triggering of AF/flutter, non-dihydropyridine group CCB (diltiazem or verapamil) (Class IIa, LOE B) or beta-blocker (metoprolol) need to be given (Class IIa, LOE C) to slow down the AV node for a long time. CCB should not be given in cases of decompensated HF or wide-complex tachycardia in adults and in young children. Likewise, concomitant use of different antiarrhythmic medications should be discouraged. Combined use of AV nodal blocking agents can cause severe bradyarrhythmias. Agents such as amiodarone, procainamide, sotalol can provide rate control in AF/flutter, and sometimes they can cause sinus rhythm. Thromboembolic complications should also be sought after conversion.

The aforementioned agents may not be beneficial in patients with PSVT triggered by preexcitation such as WPW or LGL, and they may trigger fatal arrhythmias by increasing the ventricular rate (Class III, LOE C). It will be correct to ask for a consultation.

4. Multifocal atrial tachycardia (MAT)

There are at least three different P wave morphologies originating from the atrium in the ECG tracks. There are also variable PP, PR and RR ranges. The heart rate is above 100 beats per minute and the rhythm is irregular. It can be mistakenly interpreted as AF. The typical patient is the elderly one with chronic lung disease such as COPD. Treatment is to correct the underlying disease. Standard antiarrhythmics are ineffective in suppressing multiple atrial ectopias and these agents may have toxic effects. Also, digoxin depresses the AV node and slows the ventricular rate. In the management, magnesium sulphate 2 g IV is given within 60 seconds; followed by administration of 1–2 g/hour with a constant infusion rate. Verapamil slows down the ventricular response with 5–10 mg IV administration, reduces ectopic stimuli in some patients, and provides conversion to sinus rhythm in many patients.

5. Atrial fibrillation: definition, recognition and treatment

Atrial fibrillation (AF) is the inactive 'worm bag-like' oscillations of the atria, which means there is no true atrium contraction. Different electrical vectors move in different directions simultaneously from the atrial myocardium, causing irregular and rapid impulses. Regular atrial activity is not recorded in AF. There are no P waves and no sawtooth/flutter waves. There are only irregular, unequal oscillations called F waves. Although the atrial rate is around 400 bpm, it is limited by the refractory period and can be very variable. The RR intervals are unequal; thus it is an irregular rhythm. Acute AF, which prompts a visit to the ED is therefore common in the emergency, is often discloses a high ventricular rate.

AF is the most common rhythm disorder encountered and managed by emergency physicians following only sinus tachycardia [4, 5]. Majority of patients with AF and atrial flutter (AFL) can be treated and discharged in the ED without the need for hospitalization. As the age increases, AF is encountered more frequently, with a male predominance.

AF can be acute or chronic. Patients with acute AF (AAF) mostly present with a rapid ventricular response, that is, more than 100 beats per minute. In chronic AF, the ventricular response can be normal, high or low (**Figure 3A** and **B**).

AAF is the term used for AF that lasted no longer than 48 hours from the onset of an attack. It is an entity triggered by many reasons; poor outcomes of AAF arise mostly due to hemodynamic instability and thromboembolic events. The most common causes are mitral valve diseases, acute coronary syndromes (ACS)/ischemic heart disease and thyrotoxicosis (**Table 2**).

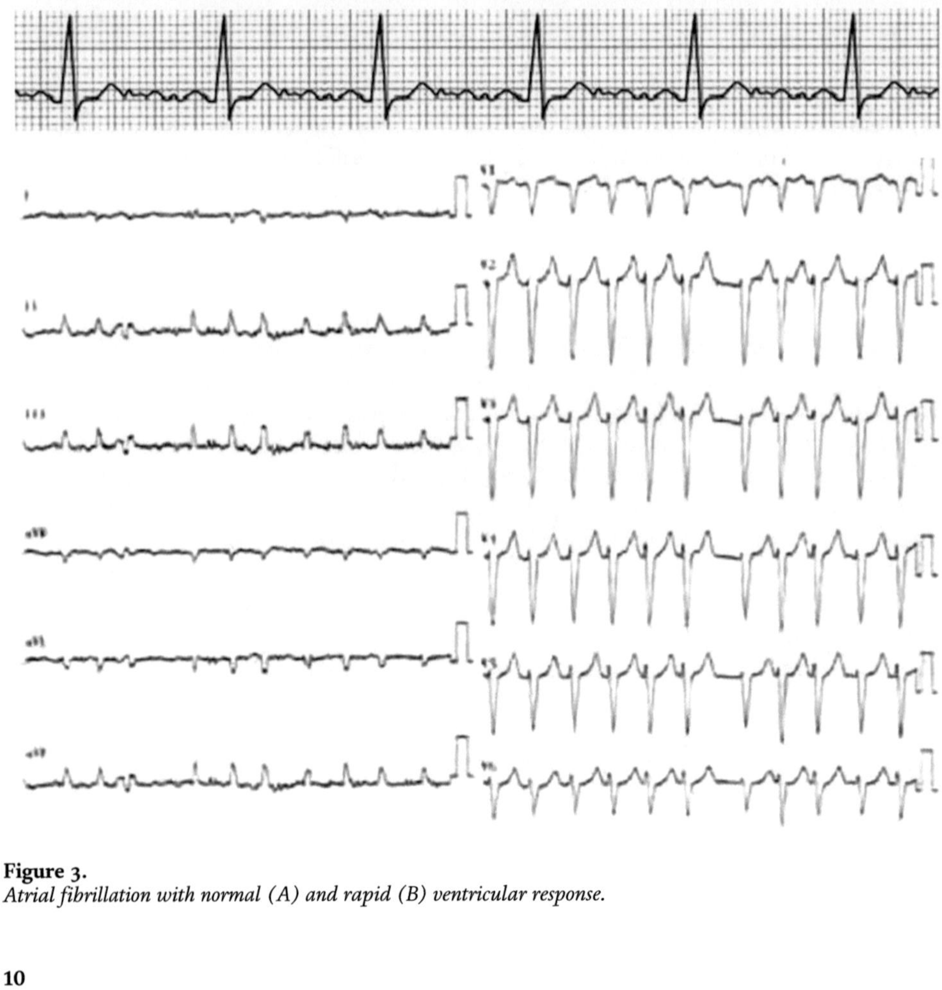

Figure 3.
Atrial fibrillation with normal (A) and rapid (B) ventricular response.

Causes that trigger AAF	Factors predisposing to acute or chronic AF
Structural cardiac abnormalities/cardiomyopathies/valvular diseases, mainly mitral	• atrial enlargement, • congestive heart failure • vagal stimulation, • atherosclerosis • hyperthyroidism • refractory period differs in various parts of the atrium.
Inflammation/infections/fever (may or may not affect the heart directly	
Fluid/electrolyte disorders, dehydration	
Strenous exercise/athletic training	
Hormonal and autonomic nervous system disorders	
ACS/atherosclerosis/coronary heart disease	
Intoxications: carbon monoxide/alcohol	
Hypoxemia	
Pulmonary embolism	
Overt release/intake of thyroid hormones	

Table 2.
Triggering causes of AAF and predisposing factors to acute or chronic AF.

In AF, HF may ensue because the heart cannot achieve pump activity as it did normally before, especially at high ventricular rates. Patients with AF are also predisposed to peripheral venous and atrial embolism with the risk of pulmonary and systemic arterial embolism. Like cancer, cardiovascular diseases including AF impose several risk factors and pathophysiologic mechanisms, including inflammation and alterations in platelet function, which ultimately result in thromboembolism [6]. Likewise, some risk factors increase tendency of AF and venous thrombosis together, such as obesity [7]. Five to 15% of patients with chronic AF can be expected to have thromboembolism once a year. Therefore, patients with chronic AF should regularly use anticoagulant medication while addressing other necessary measures to mitigate any other risk factors for thromboembolism.

6. Clinical status

Hemodynamic stability and recognition of factors which precipitate the arrhythmia are to be addressed at first. The onset of rhythm disorder should be especially questioned with special regard to acute/chronic distinction. It should be treated as chronic AF and the presence of thrombi should be ruled out if the clinician is not persuaded that it is an acute/*de novo* attack. Stroke risk should be evaluated with validated scores.

In patients with AAF a pulse rate of around 180 bpm which may cause instability, is recorded frequently, and in rare cases, it may pose a danger by exceeding 200 bpm.

In cases with Wolff-Parkinson-White (WPW) syndrome, which has an aberrant conduction pathway, extremely high heart rates can be life-threatening as a result of by-passed AV node [8].

Approximately half of the patients presenting with AAF return to sinus rhythm within 48 hours. This rule is especially true for those whose etiology is highlighted, and treatment is commenced.

AF frequently accompanies hypertension. In contrary developed countries, AF is also common in the setting of rheumatic heart diseases, especially with mitral stenosis in developing countries. Loss of atrial contractions, especially in cases of left ventricular failure, may lead to the acute exacerbation or worsening of HF.

Common complaints in patients with AF are fatigue, palpitations, chest pain, and shortness of breath. The reason for this is that the ejection fraction is reduced due to AF. Another important consequence of AF is that it predisposes to stroke and peripheral acute artery occlusions as a result of the formation of atrial thrombi. Troponin-positive coronary artery disease was detected in 5% of the patients who presented to the ED with AAF. Acute-onset AF, especially, should be considered ACS until proven otherwise. Thromboembolic disease is a major complication of AF and must be ruled out in every patient with AF. Five to 15% of these patients experience embolic/ischemic stroke every year.

Differential diagnosis of AAF includes entities such as AFL, PSVT, sinus rhythm, and AV nodal tachycardia [9]. These diseases can be easily differentiated from each other basically both with their clinical features and their ECGs.

6.1 Clinical distinction

Unlike the clinical features of AAF outlined above, PSVT cases describe the onset of the arrhythmia very clearly. Most of the cases have gained experience and are knowledgeable about CSM, Valsalva manoeuver, and rhythm correcting agents, and some even present to the ED only after failing to treat themselves with manoeuvers. Its findings are more stable, serious findings are rarely detected. Pharmacological cardioversion (PCV) with agents such as metoprolol and diltiazem is generally uneventful. Of these, verapamil is used less frequently than before, due to its side effect profile. Electrical cardioversion (ECV) is required in a small group, ECV can be applied with low doses such as 50 J.

Patients with AFL (flutter) can notice that the attack has started more clearly than those with AF, and they tend to come to the ED more acutely and a worse condition can be noted. It may accompany acute coronary syndromes including AMI and unstable angina pectoris. Therefore, these patients present with chest pain, dyspnea and hypotension more commonly in this group, compared to AF. The ventricular rate, or pulse rate, changes according to the degree of AV block, which directly affects the clinical status and stability. Since the atrial rate is generally around 300 bpm, the ventricular rate is often recorded as 75, 100 or 150 bpm, which exactly correspond to 1:2, 1:3, 1:4 blocks. For ECV, 30–50 J with monophasic defibrillators is usually sufficient.

Multifocal atrial tachycardia (MAT) is mostly seen in advanced stages of chronic lung diseases and critical HF. It has also been reported in cases of theophylline poisoning and those who consume caffeine excessively. Atrial rhythm is usually between 100 and 180 bpm. ECV is not indicated in this entity.

Differential diagnosis by ECG:

In a patient whose clinic is suitable for the diagnosis of MAT, at least three different P wave structures and variable P–P, P-R, and R-R intervals are sought in the ECG tracing. In AFL, at around 300 atrial velocities, regular waves called saw tooth (seesaw), characterized by the absence of isoelectric line, are seen. Findings are best observed in limb leads II, III, and aVF.

The presence of fibrillation (f) waves replacing the isoelectric line in the ECG in patients with AF, the absence of a consistent and continuously traceable P wave, are observed as 'irregular' rhythm characterized by the inequality of R-R intervals. As a rule, QRS waves are normal, that is, narrow. Delta waves and short PR should be investigated for concomitant WPW syndrome.

7. Imaging and laboratory

The purpose of imaging in AAF cases under emergency conditions is to collect information about differential diagnoses and triggering causes, and more importantly, to anticipate and prevent thromboembolic events.

There are no 'routine' laboratory examinations to be ordered in every case of AF, instead, a cost-effective list of workup can be culminated for each individual patient. For example, pulmonary embolism can be distinguished by POCUS-computed tomography-angiography. Other diseases associated with or triggering AF can be sought for via chest radiography; findings compatible with pneumonia, congestive heart failure, enlargement of the heart chambers, chronic pericarditis, aneurysm can be investigated. Carboxyhaemoglobin (COHb) level is critical in guiding the treatment in cases where carbon monoxide poisoning is thought to be the trigger for AAF attack. ECG, troponin and creatine kinase levels can yield vital findings in terms of acute ischemic heart disease. Haemoglobin and haematocrit should be requested in terms of acute haemorrhagic losses, blood urea nitrogen and creatinine levels should be requested for uremic pericarditis or RF. Oxygenation should be measured under emergency conditions with pulse oximetry, hypoxemia should be excluded and corrected, if any. In cases such as diabetic ketoacidosis or COPD, arterial blood gas analysis should be used.

In a recent study, it has been reported that patients with NT-proBNP levels below 450 pg./ml mostly reverted to sinus rhythm during their hospital stay, whereas patients with values above 1800 pg./ml are found to have persistent AF [10]. For this reason, BNP levels need to be requested in patients with dyspnea, in order to distinguish between heart failure and lung disease. If thyroid diseases such as thyrotoxicosis, Basedow-Graves' disease, multinodular goitere are considered as triggering causes, T3, T4 and thyroid stimulating hormone levels will be useful.

It is vital to exclude pericardial tamponade due to trauma and patients with suspected cardiac arrest (asystole or pulseless electrical activity) despite the electrical activity on the ECG under emergency conditions. In addition, POCUS/echocardiography evaluates the size and motion of the heart chambers, the presence of a heart-related mass, valve problems and the presence of intracardiac thrombus. In this way, important information can be obtained with a low-cost, simple application at the bedside.

The most important limitation of the technique is that its reliability and accuracy are dependent on the experience and ability of the operator. Since the results can also change with the position that can be given to the patient, there is a limitation in cases who cannot easily change position or those with obesity.

For ideal cardiac USG/POCUS, lowering the pulse is important. For this, depending on the condition of the patient with atrial tachyarrhythmia, beta-blocker or calcium channel blocker agents can be used.

Beta-blockers (metoprolol) may be preferred in young people with anxiety, coronary artery disease or hyperthyroidism, and calcium channel blockers in other groups and in patients who are contraindicated to beta-blockers such as asthma. PO/IV metoprolol should be preferred for beta blockade and IV esmolol in more urgent cases. Diltiazem, one of the calcium channel blockers, is the first choice due to its more positive side effect profile than verapamil. Concomitant administration of metoprolol and calcium channel blocker in selected cases is acceptable, but attention should be paid to dose adjustment and titration to effect.

Echocardiography can be performed by transesophageal (TEE) or transthoracic (TTE) methods in patients with AF. Since TEE is performed using the oesophageal probe, it both takes images from the window closer to the heart anatomically and gives a more accurate result as it eliminates the blocking effect of the chest and ribs. However, in some cases, it is difficult to tolerate and may take longer. TTE is a faster diagnostic tool chosen under emergency conditions. TEE is more sensitive in showing the left atrium, left atrial appendix (LAA), atrial septum, and aortic arch. For example, potential sources of cardiac embolism that may be overlooked by TTE in stroke cases can be determined by TEE.

The cause of cardiac embolism can be found in nearly 80% of the cases with TEE in patients with an uncertain cause of stroke. With TTE, this rate is lower, between 15 and 40%. TTE is often chosen in elderly patients with a known cardioembolic cause. TEE yields better results in patients under 50 years of age for whom the cause of stroke cannot be determined.

In a detailed echocardiographic examination to be performed in patients with AF, hemodynamic variables such as mean diastolic mitral gradient, pulmonary artery pressure, mitral valve area, tricuspid and mitral regurgitation, left atrial diameter should be measured and given quantitatively. In addition, the Wilkins mitral valve score is calculated. For example, in different studies, the mitral valve score and tricuspid valve involvement among those with mitral stenosis were found to be higher in patients with AF than those with sinus rhythm, indicating the prevalence of rheumatic activity [11].

Echocardiographic findings are closely related to the clinical course. For example, in studies examining the variables that affect the conversion of AF cases to sinus rhythm, the duration of AF attack less than 24 hours, young age, left atrial diameter and absence of primary heart disease appear as independent variables. Doğan et al. found only the duration of AF as an effective factor in conversion [12]. In this study, the mean left atrium diameter of patients presenting with AF was found to be 39.0 mm.

In recent years, after correction of AF with ECV, attention has been drawn to the 'stunning' phenomenon and related TTE findings have been underlined. Decreased LAA flow rates, decreased LAA discharge fraction, decreased transmitral inflow rates, and the appearance of spontaneous echo contrast has been reported as findings indicating atrial stunning.

8. Contemporary management of AAF in the acute setting

In cases presenting with AAF, the treatment of the underlying disease, eliminating pain and anxiety, providing oxygenation and correcting the hemodynamics are primary and mandatory goals to achieve. After this treatment, a return to sinus rhythm can be accomplished without any other intervention in most cases.

Apart from this basic principle, there are three mainstays in the treatment of AF cases.

1. Provision of normal sinus rhythm and maintaining its stability,
2. Although AF is not terminated, reducing the heart rate to a normal/acceptable level
3. Prevention of formation of mural thrombi (besides ACS, some malignancies, aneurysm etc. can also lead to a tendency of thrombus formation)

8.1 Pearl

If rapid ventricular rate AAF is accompanied by rate-related symptoms (HF, pulmonary edema, dyspnea, impaired consciousness, ischemic chest pain), rate control should be provided immediately. As with flutter, agents such as diltiazem, verapamil or beta blocker (propranolol or metoprolol) can be used. ECV should be considered in those with acute hemodynamic compromise.

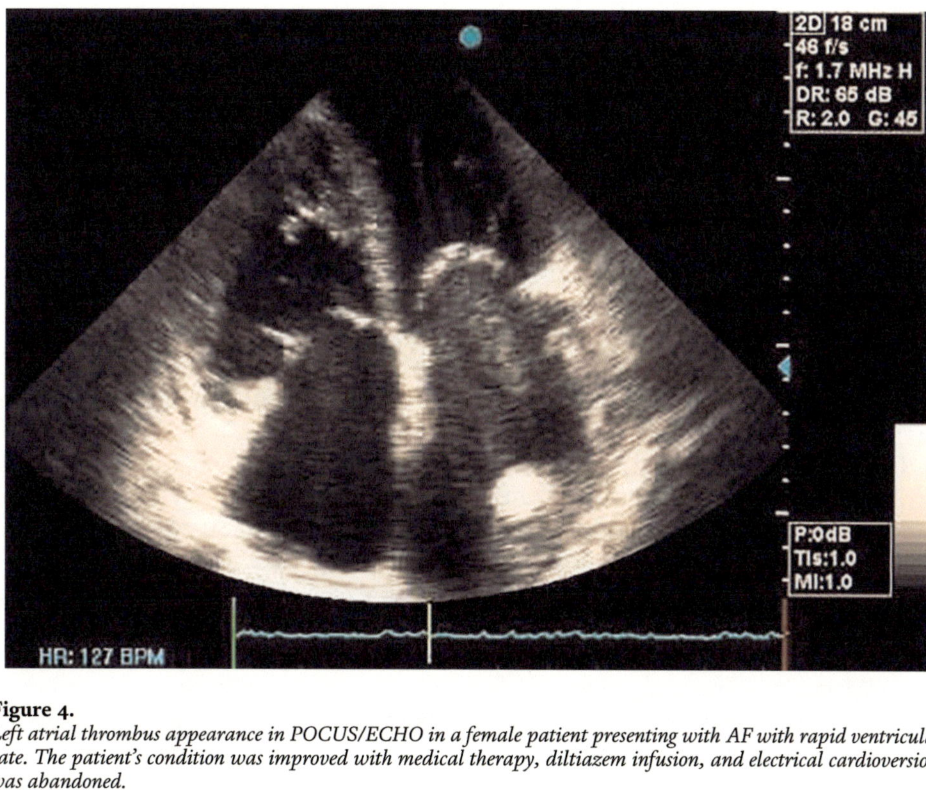

Figure 4.
Left atrial thrombus appearance in POCUS/ECHO in a female patient presenting with AF with rapid ventricular rate. The patient's condition was improved with medical therapy, diltiazem infusion, and electrical cardioversion was abandoned.

When AAF cases are considered to be hemodynamically stable, one of two ways is chosen in treatment. These two options, known as rhythm control or rate control, are selected and applied in accord with the patient's clinical characteristics. Stiell et al. in their population-based study in Canada examined whether the methods conducted in different centres differed from each other [4]. It was observed that the rhythm control strategy was applied to approximately 60% of 1018 AAF and AFL cases, and ECV was performed primarily for 40% of them. In total, 83% of the patients were discharged from the ED successfully. The variables that affect the choice of rhythm control strategy and the decision of ECV independently from other factors were determined as age, previous ECV history, presence of HF, and the centre admitted the patient (**Figure 4**).

In general, treatment strategies can be divided into conservative (preparation for elective ECV after speed control and anticoagulation) and aggressive (performing cardioversion as ECV or chemical/pharmacological cardioversion (PCV) in appropriate patients under safety precautions in the ED). It has been reported that there are important differences between physicians and disciplines in terms of approach to AAF.

9. Rhythm control and cardioversion (conversion to sinus rhythm)

ECV or PCV can be applied under emergency conditions to provide the conversion of AAF to sinus rhythm. The difference between cardioversion performed under emergency conditions and elective procedure is that the rhythm is returned to normal without anticoagulation in emergency practice, whereas in an elective procedure, it would be clarified that there is no thrombus and other contraindications are excluded, and the cardioversion procedure is performed.

Therefore, it should be ensured as much as possible that less than 48 hours have passed from the onset of AAF for ECV and that the patient does not pose a high risk for embolic stroke [5]. If you cannot be sure how long has passed, a rate control strategy should be adopted at first. Therapeutic anticoagulation should be commenced in these cases 3 weeks before and 4 weeks following ECV. However, in the case of unplanned cardioversion, AHA and ESC guidelines agree that cardioversion can be performed after an echocardiographic examination for thrombus exclusion [13]. Canadian Cardiology Society guidelines recommend that in patients with AF lasting for 12–48 hours, transesophageal echocardiography (TEE) is solely abdicable in patients with a low risk of stroke (CHADS2-score: 0–1). Since the duration of AF does not necessarily correlate with the occurrence of thrombi and AF-onset is often unsure, low-risk TOE prior to cardioversion should be employed [14].

In a very recent study, Bellone et al. randomized 247 patients into these two groups (ECV vs. PCV) [15]. The success rate of ECV was higher (89 vs. 73%). The mean time period spent in the ED is also much shorter in the ECV group (180 vs. 420 minutes). Side effects and adverse events occurred in a short time and in very small subgroups. Similarly, Cristoni et al. published a study in 2010, which showed that by establishing a short observation unit linked with the ED, these cases could be effectively treated without the need for hospitalization [16]. In this study, they were randomized to ECV (n = 171) and PCV (n = 151) groups, and discharge in sinus rhythm was achieved in 93 and 51%, respectively. During the 6-month follow-up, two patients in the ECV group had stroke. As a result, the treatment of AAF cases can be safely performed by applying ECV in the short observation unit.

More than 60% of patients return to normal sinus rhythm with 100 J and more than 80% with 200 J. ECV will benefit the patient only if the precipitating event is resolved. Therefore, ECV is only an emergency solution to save time (**Table 3**).

Drugs used in PCV are predominantly Class IC and III, according to Vaughan-Williams classification. Recently, Conti et al. reported that flecainide, propafenone or amiodarone were administered to a total of 378 patients in a non-randomized design for PCV in the Italian Eds, and 87% of the total group returned to sinus rhythm within 6 hours [17]. The success rates of the three drugs were 72, 55 and 30%, respectively ($p < 0.001$). Conversion times were also sorted by the same sequence, with an average of 178, 292 and 472 minutes ($p < 0.001$). They postulated that IC group antiarrhythmics (flecainide, propafenone) are apparently more efficacious than Class III drugs (amiodarone) and should be selected first for PCV. Propafenone 150 mg tablets, which are commercially available in most places from the IC group, can be administered orally as 300 or 600 mg. We can safely point out that PCV can be safely and successfully administered in the ED.

In a Croatian study, it has been reported that a success rate close to 100% has been achieved via PCV by administering three drugs from different pharmacological classes consecutively within a certain protocol [18].

Class I agents that produce antiarrhythmic effects by blocking sodium channels are divided into groups IA, IB and IC. Class IC drugs are one of the groups with the highest potential to terminate AAF via PCV. Propafenone, which is frequently used for this purpose in many centres, is also in this group. It should be selected in young patients with AF without structural heart disease. Bradycardia and heart failure, which can be life-threatening, can be seen rarely with this agent.

Although amiodarone (Class III; blocking sodium and potassium channels) is one of the most effective antiarrhythmic agents, it is less effective in the termination of

ESC	AHA/ACC/HRS	CCS
Favouring rhythm control:		
• First AF episode or short history	• Symptoms under rate control	• Highly symptomatic or significant Quality of life (QoL) impairment
• Younger age	• Younger age	• Recently diagnosed (<1 year)
• Arrhythmia induced cardiomyopathy	• First AF episode	• Multiple recurrences
• No or few comorbidities/heart disease	• Arrhythmia induced cardiomyopathy	• Difficulty to achieve rate control
• Normal to moderate increased Left atrial volume-index.(LAVI)/atrial conduction delay (limited atrial remodelling)	• Patient's choice	• Arrhythmia induced cardiomyopathy
• Rate control difficult to achieve	• Arrhythmia induced cardiomyopathy	
• AF precipitated by a temporary event	• Failed rate control	
• Patient's choice		

Table 3.
ESC, AHA/ACC/HRS and CCS guidelines on indications for rhythm control.

AAF by PCV. A feature that does not exist in other drugs is that it can be used safely in individuals with the poor general condition, the elderly and/or those with underlying structural heart disease.

9.1 Use of amiodarone for PCV

IV: Infused primarily 150 mg/10 minutes. Then 1 mg/min is infused for 6 hours, 0.5 mg/min for 18 hours. The maximum total dose is 10 g. It can be continued orally (100–200 mg/day).

> Can the patients terminate AF themselves? Yes. One approach that can also be seen as a variant of the rhythm control strategy is that individuals with infrequent attacks are given a certain training, and these individuals immediately receive PCV by taking the appropriate medication right next to them. This approach, also known as the 'drug in the pocket' concept, can be used very beneficially in selected patient groups.

Flecainide (95%) and ibutilide (76%) were found to be the most effective drugs used for PCV in 376 patients with AAF in the ED [19]. Amiodarone, digoxin and diltiazem have very low success rates. A striking result is an observation that patients presenting with low blood pressure and who had a short period of time from the onset of AF to treatment revert to sinus rhythm with higher success.

9.2 Procedure recommendation

For PCV, propafenone from group IC can be used for conversion of AF to NSR. For this purpose, 600 mg propafenone (4 × 150 mg tb) is administered orally at a time and the patient is expected to convert within a few hours. This procedure is only recommended in the hospital.

ECG monitoring is recommended because a prolonged period of asystole, rarely syncope or prolonged bradyarrhythmias may occur during 'successful' conversion.

Medication	Starting dose (adult ~70 kg)	Dose/kg (for titration)	Duration of effect	Side effect
Midazolam (for sedation, anxiolysis)	1–2 mg IV	0.04–0.06 mg/kg (IV/IM)	60–90 minutes	Respiratory depression, hypotension (very rare at recommended doses)
Etomidate (for sedation, anxiolysis)	15–20 mg IV	0.2–0.3 mg/kg IV	20–30 minutes	Myoclonus, adrenocortical suppression in long-term administration
Fentanyl (for analgesia)	1–2 mcg/kg IV	0.5–1.0 mcg/kg IV	1–2 hours	Respiratory depression, chest rigidity (very rare at recommended doses)
Naloxone (narcotic antagonist)	0.2–0.4 mg IV (up to 2 mg)	0.4 mg IV	2–3 hours	Tachycardia

Table 4.
Sedatives and narcotics, doses, duration of action and expected side effects for sedoanalgesia used in ECV procedure in the ED. the drugs are used by an experienced emergency physician or anaesthesiologist, titrated with respect to the response of the patient.

10. Synchronized/simultaneous cardioversion

When midazolam and fentanyl are administered at recommended doses and under appropriate conditions, the side effect profile is at an acceptable level (**Table 4**). In the presence of signs of opioid overdose that may occur, albeit very rarely, naloxone should be used by titrating at the recommended doses in the table. Ketamine, which is widely used for sedoanalgesia in other indications, is not preferred in this group of cases as it may have tachycardic effects.

11. Rate control

Rate control strategy is a treatment approach preferred in patients with AF attacks thought to recur especially in those with structural heart disease, coronary artery disease, and advanced age. It is aimed to improve the symptoms by reducing the heart rate. Patients who are not selected/unsuitable for ECV are evaluated in the rate control group.

Antiarrhythmic agents such as beta-blockers (metoprolol), calcium channel blockers (diltiazem), and amiodarone are widely used for rate control. The serious toxic effects of amiodarone on many organs and systems limit its use. Digoxin is also a frequently used agent in the past, but it is rarely recommended in contemporary practice.

IV beta-blocker and nondihydropyridine CCB (diltiazem) is the drug of choice for acute rate control in AF with rapid ventricular response (Class IIa, LOE A).

Digoxin and amiodarone can be used for rate control in patients with CHF + AF. However, after the use of amiodarone, the risk of return to sinus rhythm and resultant embolization should be taken into account.

A large complex, irregularly irregular rhythm may reflect an AF with pre-excitation (WPW/LGL). Expert consultation should be obtained early.

- Adenosine, CCB, digoxin and β-blocking agents that cause AV nodal block should be avoided, as they pose a risk of increasing the ventricular rate.
- These cases are often converted to NSR with emergency ECV. If this is unavailable, other than above mentioned objectionable agents can be tried.

Procainamide is a widely used agent in most parts of the world for PCV. In a study in which the 'Ottawa Aggressive Protocol' put forward in Canada in the last decade was tested, 660 AAF (4.9% AFL) cases were taken as a cohort [20]. If it could not be understood whether the AAF attack lasted longer than 48 hours, the presence of mural thrombus was examined by TEE. Initially, IV procainamide was given to all cases, and a conversion rate of 58.3% was achieved. ECV procedure was performed in all remaining 243 cases, it was successful in 91.7% of them. Recurrent attacks were observed in 8.6% of the cases within 7 days. The patients stayed in the ED for an average of 4.9 hours (3.9 hours in patients with PCV, 6.5 hours in patients with ECV) and 96.8% were discharged from the ED.

12. Antithrombotic-antiaggregant treatment in patients with AF

In AF cases in which effective contractions do not occur, blood may undergo stasis and turn into clots, especially in the left atrium. This phenomenon is clearly seen in AF patients lasting for 48 hours and older. The delivery of these clots to the arterial circulation via the aorta occurs most often during the conversion of AAF to normal sinus rhythm, so it is important to demonstrate that there is no clot for ECV/PCV of chronic AF. Arterial circulation may stop in any part of the body with this event called thromboembolism of mural thrombi. Apart from AF, cancer, haematological problems, coronary artery disease, heart failure and ventricular aneurysms can pave the way to thrombus formation. Acute arterial occlusion, renal infarction, acute mesenteric embolism may occur, but the most important morbidity is that it causes cerebral thromboembolism or stroke.

Warfarin (Coumadine) and heparin are agents that prevent fibrin formation, they are in the anticoagulant group. Acetyl salicylic acid (ASA, Aspirin) and clopidogrel (Plavix) or ticagrelor (Brilinta) are antiaggregant or antiplatelet agents. The combined use of P2Y12 inhibitor and ASA is called dual antiplatelet treatment (DAPT). Among these, warfarin prevents clot formation in the most efficient way, provides full effectiveness within a few days after its use, and requires monitoring with prothrombin time (PT) and international normalized ratio (INR) level every 4–8 weeks. In recent years, the 'triple antiplatelet therapy' (TAPT) method has been in question, with the addition of an agent from the DOAC group (such as dabigatran/rivaroxaban) to the DAPT regimen. Recent reports pointed out that TAPT strategy may be associated with higher bleeding episodes and mortality compared to a DAPT regimen—the combination of an anticoagulant and a P2Y12 inhibitor [21].

As of the update in January 2019, the following recommendations are in effect: [22].

- If the CHA2DS2-VASc score is > = 2 in AF + ACS cases, warfarin (vitamin K antagonist-VKA) 'triple therapy/triple therapy' (TAPT) is recommended in addition to the DAPT (aspirin + P2Y12 inhibitor) regimen.
- Double therapy in the form of warfarin (vitamin K antagonist) with P2Y12 inhibitor + dose adjustment after stenting is an acceptable treatment.
- P2Y12 inhibitor (clopidogrel or ticagrelor) + oral anticoagulant rivaroxaban, dabigatran or VKA with dose adjustment can be given as an alternative.

13. Does AF in my patient cause a cerebrovascular accident?

Yes, it can. In NVAF, the CHA2DS2-VASc score and risk criteria have been used in recent years instead of the CHADS2 criteria in 2001 in order to predict this more clearly (**Tables 5** and **6**).

Score	CHA2DS2-VASc risk criteria
1	CHF
1	Hypertension
2	Age ≥ 75
1	Diabetes mellitus
2	Stroke/TIA/thromboembolic event
1	Vascular disease (MI, PAH, aortic disease)
1	Age 65–74 years
1	Woman

Table 5.
CHA2DS2-VASc score and risk criteria.

CHA2DS2-VASc score	Annual stroke risk (%, per year)	Recommendation
0	0	No treatment
1	1.3	No treatment or aspirin or OAC
2	2.2	OAC
3	3.2	
4	4.0	
5	6.7	
6	9.8	
7	9.6	
8	6.7	
9	15.2	

Table 6.
CHA2DS2-VASc score and annual stroke risks with relevant treatment recommendations.

14. How is emergency anticoagulation done before ECV?

If PCV or ECV is planned in a patient with AF that is thought to last longer than 48 hours, one of the following three regimens should be started:

- emergency IV (unfractionated) heparin (target PTT, 60 seconds)
- or LMWH (enoxaparin 0.5 mg/kg or 40 mg once or twice daily)
- or VKA/warfarin for at least 5 days (target INR, 2.5).

When no thrombus is seen and ECV/PCV is successful, anticoagulation is continued for another 4 weeks (target INR, 2.5). If a thrombus is seen, ECV/PCV is delayed. TEE should be repeated before each ECV attempt.

At the earliest period in a hemodynamically unstable case with a suspected ECV

- emergency IV (unfractionated) heparin (target PTT, 60 seconds)
- or LMWH (at DVT therapeutic dose) should be initiated.

After successful cardioversion, VKA/warfarin (target INR, 2.5) is continued for at least 4 weeks. Long-term anticoagulation will depend on the patient's risk status, previous cardioversion procedures or another embolism status. For example, maintenance with rivaroxaban, one of the NOACs, is more suitable for those who have had a pulmonary embolism.

The above regimens are also valid in cases with flutter (Grade 2C).

The following agents were found to be effective in cases where treatment with OAC was considered:

- Warfarin (with the target INR in the range of 2–3)
- Dabigatran
- Rivaroxaban

Variable				**Score**
Hypertension				1
Renal failure (dialysis, transplant, creatinine >2.26 mg/dL or 200 μmol/L)				1
Liver disease (cirrhosis or bilirubin >2x normal + AST/ALT/ALP > 3x normal)				1
A history of stroke				1
A previous history of significant bleeding from any area				1
Labile INR (unstable/high INR, time within the therapeutic range < 60%)				1
Age > 65				1
Use of drugs such as aspirin, clopidogrel, NSAID that may cause bleeding tendency				1
Alcohol use (≥8 times a week)				1
HAS-BLED score	Risk group	Major bleeding risk (%)	Percentage of pts. with a bleeding annually	Recommendation
0	Low	0.9	1.13	
1		3.4	1.02	Anticoagulation can be considered
2	Moderate	4.1	1.88	Anticoagulation can be considered
3	High	5.8	3.72	Alternatives for anticoagulation can be considered
4		8.9	8.70	
5		9.1	12.50	
>5	Very high	—	—	Think about individualized options

Table 7.
HAS-BLED score.

- Apixaban
- Edoxaban

15. I am treating the patient with OAC. Do I cause a bleed in the patient?

Yes, there is a risk of bleeding. HAS-BLED score is the best tool developed for this (**Table 7**). This term acronym consists of the initials of the criteria 'Hypertension, Abnormal liver/renal function, Stroke history, Bleeding predisposition, Labile INR, Elderly, Drug/alcohol usage'.

16. Conclusion and summary

SVT AF represents a costly public health problem due to its high prevalence and high morbidity attributed to the disease itself and inherent complications. It causes serious consequences through hemodynamic complications and thromboembolic problems such as stroke and acute arterial occlusion. POCUS/echocardiography is vital in patients with AF because it shows potential thromboembolism at its source and also reveals cardiac functions, valve and chamber problems. Safe and effective pharmacological or electrical cardioversion (PCV/ECV) are current treatments of choice in cases with acute AF while selected cases will be candidates for rate control strategy. BB, CCB, adenosine, amiodarone and propafenone are among the most commonly used agents in this regard. There is not a standard regimen to apply to every case, but specific agents need to be selected in regard to the patient and the situation.

Author details

Özgür Karcıoğlu
Department of Emergency Medicine, University of Health Sciences, Taksim Training and Research Hospital, Istanbul, Turkey

*Address all correspondence to: okarcioglu@gmail.com

References

[1] Lip GYH, Watson T. Atrial fibrillation (acute onset). Clinical Evidence. 2006; **15**:1-3

[2] Smith GD, Fry MM, Taylor D, Morgans A, Cantwell K. Effectiveness of the Valsalva manoeuvre for reversion of supraventricular tachycardia. Cochrane Database of Systematic Reviews. 2015; **2015**(2):CD009502. DOI: 10.1002/14651858.CD009502.pub3

[3] Brugada J, Katritsis DG, Arbelo E, et al. 2019 ESC guidelines for the management of patients with supraventricular tachycardia. The task force for the management of patients with supraventricular tachycardia of the European Society of Cardiology (ESC). European Heart Journal. 2020;**41**(5): 655-720. DOI: 10.1093/eurheartj/ehz467

[4] Stiell IG, Macle L, CCS Atrial Fibrillation Guidelines Committee. Canadian cardiovascular society atrial fibrillation guidelines 2010: Management of recent-onset atrial fibrillation and flutter in the emergency department. The Canadian Journal of Cardiology. 2011;**27**(1):38-46

[5] Stiell IG, Birnie D. Managing recent-onset atrial fibrillation in the emergency department. Annals of Emergency Medicine. 2011;**57**(1):31-32

[6] Leiva O, Abdel Hameid D, Connors JM, Cannon CP, Bhatt DL. Common pathophysiology in cancer, atrial fibrillation, atherosclerosis, and thrombosis. JACC: CardioOncology. 2021;**3**(5):619-634. DOI: 10.1016/j.jaccao.2021.08.011

[7] Nasser MF, Jabri A, Gandhi S, Rader F. Oral anticoagulant use in morbid obesity and post bariatric surgery: A review. The American Journal of Medicine. 2021;**134**(12):1465-1475. DOI: 10.1016/j.amjmed.2021.07.017

[8] Fengler BT, Brady WJ, Plautz CU. Atrial fibrillation in the Wolff-Parkinson-white syndrome: ECG recognition and treatment in the ED. The American Journal of Emergency Medicine. 2007;**25**(5):576-583

[9] Thomas D, Eckardt L, Estner HL, et al. Typisches Vorhofflattern: Diagnostik und Therapie [typical atrial flutter: Diagnosis and therapy]. Germanica. 2016;**27**(1):46-56

[10] Buccelletti F, Gilardi E, Marsiliani D, Carroccia A, Silveri NG, Franceschi F. Predictive value of NT-proBNP for cardioversion in a new onset atrial fibrillation. European Journal of Emergency Medicine. 2011;**18**(3):157-161

[11] Kabukçu M, Arslantas E, Ates I, Demircioglu F, Ersel F. Clinical, echocardiographic, and hemodynamic characteristics of rheumatic mitral valve stenosis and atrial fibrillation. Angiology. 2005;**56**(2):159-163. DOI: 10.1177/000331970505600206

[12] Doğan A, Ergene O, Nazli C, et al. Yeni Atrial Fibrilasyonda Kendiliğinden Sonlanma Belirleyicileri ve Propafenon ile Uzun Süreli Sinüs Ritminin İdamesi. Türk Kardiyoloji Derneği Arşivi. 2003; **31**:392-399

[13] Wolfes J, Ellermann C, Frommeyer G, Eckardt L. Evidence-based treatment of atrial fibrillation around the globe: Comparison of the latest ESC, AHA/ACC/HRS, and CCS guidelines on the management of atrial fibrillation. Reviews in Cardiovascular Medicine. 2022;**23**:56

[14] Hilberath JN, Oakes DA, Shernan SK, Bulwer BE, D'Ambra MN,

Eltzschig HK. Safety of transesophageal echocardiography. Journal of the American Chemical Society. 2010;**23**: 1115-1127

[15] Bellone A, Etteri M, Vettorello M, et al. Cardioversion of acute atrial fibrillation in the emergency department: A prospective randomised trial. Emergency Medicine Journal. 2012; **29**(3):188-191

[16] Cristoni L, Tampieri A, Mucci F, et al. Cardioversion of acute atrial fibrillation in the short observation unit: Comparison of a protocol focused on electrical cardioversion with simple antiarrhythmic treatment. Emergency Medicine Journal. 2011;**28**(11):932-937

[17] Conti A, Del Taglia B, Mariannini Y, et al. Management of patients with acute atrial fibrillation in the ED. The American Journal of Emergency Medicine. 2010;**28**(8):903-910

[18] Milicevic G, Gavranovic Z, Bakula M, Pazur V, Frank B. Successful conversion of recent-onset atrial fibrillation by sequential administration of up to three antiarrhythmic drugs. Clinical Cardiology. 2008;**31**(10): 472-477

[19] Hirschl MM, Wollmann C, Globits S. A 2-year survey of treatment of acute atrial fibrillation in an ED. The American Journal of Emergency Medicine. 2011; **29**(5):534-540

[20] Stiell IG, Clement CM, Perry JJ, et al. Association of the Ottawa Aggressive Protocol with rapid discharge of emergency department patients with recent-onset atrial fibrillation or flutter. CJEM. 2010;**12**(3):181-191

[21] Hussain A, Minhas A, Sarwar U, Tahir H. Triple antithrombotic therapy (triple therapy) after percutaneous coronary intervention in chronic anticoagulation: A literature review. Cureus. 2022;**14**(2):e21810. DOI: 10.7759/cureus.21810

[22] Kirolos I, Ifedili I, Maturana M, et al. Ticagrelor or prasugrel vs. clopidogrel in combination with anticoagulation for treatment of acute coronary syndrome in patients with atrial fibrillation. Annals of Translational Medicine. 2019;**7**(17):406

Chapter 2

Predictors of Atrial Fibrillation Recurrence after Ablation

Kohei Sawasaki

Abstract

Various treatment methods have been used for atrial fibrillation (AF), which has long been a cause of cerebral infarction and heart failure. Antiarrhythmic drug, the first developed treatment, was not effective in maintaining sinus rhythm and did not improve prognosis. In contrast, pulmonary vein (PV) isolation is effective in paroxysmal AF, expected to maintain sinus rhythm by 70–80% in the first session. Therefore, catheter ablation is the first-line treatment for patients with drug-resistant paroxysmal AF. For PV isolation, radiofrequency ablation was developed first, followed by cryoballoon ablation, which was shown to be not inferior to radiofrequency ablation. In contrast, for persistent AF, PV isolation alone has been found to result in a low rate of maintenance of sinus rhythm. However, there has been no impact of the additional radiofrequency application on AF recurrence rate. Recently, a number of the predictive factors of AF recurrence after AF ablation have been reported. Among them, AF duration, defibrillation threshold, left atrial volume are considered useful as predictors of atrial fibrillation recurrence after ablation. In order to improve the outcome of AF ablation, it is desirable to select patients with AF in consideration of the predictive factors of AF recurrence after AF ablation.

Keywords: atrial fibrillation, catheter ablation, pulmonary vein isolation, atrial fibrillation recurrence, defibrillation threshold

1. Introduction

Atrial fibrillation (AF), the most common sustained cardiac arrhythmia, causes cerebral infarction or heart failure. For this reason, treatment strategies for it have been studied for several years. The Atrial Fibrillation Follow-up Investigation of Rhythm Management study [1] published in 2002 reported that, compared with a rate control strategy, a rhythm control–induced strategy with medications does not help improve AF prognosis. In contrast, in catheter ablation, a nonpharmacological therapy for AF reported in 1998 by Haïssaguerre et al. [2], frequent ectopic beats arising from the pulmonary veins (PVs) contribute to AF development, while PV electrical isolation can maintain sinus rhythm. The Catheter Ablation vs. Antiarrhythmic Drug Therapy for Atrial Fibrillation (CABANA) trial [3] showed that AF recurrence occurred less frequently in the ablation group than in the standard medical therapy group. The ablation group in the same trial showed improved quality of life among patients with AF compared with the standard medical therapy group. Furthermore, the Catheter Ablation for Atrial Fibrillation with Heart Failure (CASTLE-AF) trial demonstrated that, among patients with congestive heart failure, ablation therapy prevented more events than medical therapy [4]. Based on the European Society of Cardiology Guidelines, catheter ablation is the first-line treatment for patients with drug-resistant paroxysmal AF. The FIRE AND ICE trial, which compared the efficacy and safety of radiofrequency ablation versus cryoballoon ablation for drug-resistant paroxysmal AF, determined that the cryoballoon ablation invented in recent years was not inferior to radiofrequency ablation [5]. However, compared with paroxysmal AF, persistent AF has a higher recurrence rate after ablation. To improve the prognosis of persistent AF, the ablation of atrial substrates, including linear ablation [6], complex fractionated atrial electrogram (CFAE) ablation [7], CARTOFINDER [8], ExTRa Mapping [9], and non-PV foci ablation [10], has been performed in addition to pulmonary vein isolation (PVI). A report of whether these procedures can further prevent AF recurrence is expected in the future.

AF development is orchestrated by many risk factors, including hypertension, overweight/obesity, dyslipidemia, diabetes, tobacco smoking, and excessive drinking [11, 12]. Thus, managing these risk factors is important for its prevention.

In addition, patient selection is considered important for improving treatment outcomes; therefore, it is necessary to identify a new index that correlates with patient prognosis.

2. Prognosis differs among ablation devices

2.1 AF recurrence rates for radiofrequency ablation versus cryoballoon ablation

Cryoballoon ablation is a procedure that involves inducing necrosis by exposing the myocardium to ultralow temperatures. PVI using cryoballoon ablation is currently performed in many medical facilities because cryoballoon ablation catheter is relatively easy to handle compared with a radiofrequency ablation catheter. Because the cryoballoon's radius cannot be adjusted, electrical isolation is difficult in some cases; therefore, it is important to confirm the locations of the PV and left atrium using preoperative computed tomography. In the FIRE AND ICE trial, the effectiveness of cryoballoon ablation was not inferior to that of conventional radiofrequency ablation, while the operating time for cryoballoon ablation was significantly shorter.

2.2 Laser balloon ablation

Laser balloon ablation enables observation of the crimped myocardium through the endoscope following balloon occlusion of the PV. Furthermore, the laser balloon enables free adjustment of the balloon size, target ablation site, and output power. The flexibility of the laser balloon allows an operator to perform a personalized PVI. One previous study reported that treatment outcomes for paroxysmal AF vary widely among patients [13]. Other studies reported the high incidence of phrenic neuropathy.

The isolation success and complication rates involve a learning curve. Laser balloon ablation is expected to have safe and good treatment outcomes if used properly.

2.3 Hot balloon ablation

In a hot balloon catheter, a compliant balloon made of polyurethane is attached to the end of the catheter, while electrodes for radiofrequency energy and a temperature sensor are placed inside the catheter. In hot balloon ablation, the administration of a contrast–saline mixture causes the balloon to fully expand to the appropriate size and then press against the tissue surrounding the PV. The balloon is heated to 70°C by energizing of the radiofrequency current in the balloon electrode. Compared with cryoballoon, the major difference of hot balloon ablation is to change the balloon size. Furthermore, hot balloon ablation is considered a relatively safe method because the temperature for tissue heating is ≤70°C. For that reason, the steam pop phenomenon does not occur. We are awaiting the results of a multicenter study of its clinical performance [14].

2.4 Pulsed field ablation

Pores in cell membranes are made using electric pulses, through which substances can enter cells, a phenomenon called electroporation. This method has been used for transformation, by which *Escherichia coli* or animal cells deliver DNA into cells; however, irreversible electroporation, which kills cells via irreversible perforation, has also been developed. The electric pulse frequency that kills cells differs among tissues. When applying the frequency to ablation, it is possible to selectively ablate the atrial muscle without affecting the tissues surrounding the blood vessels, nerves, and esophagus. Although the number of cases is small, the effectiveness and safety of pulsed field ablation have been reported [15].

3. AF recurrence after persistent AF ablation

Along with the progress of catheter ablation, the proportion of patients cured of AF among those with paroxysmal AF is high in all medical facilities; however, in terms of the ablation of persistent AF, the proportion of patients cured of AF still shows great variability among medical facilities.

According to the CASTLE-AF trial, catheter ablation for AF complicated by heart failure significantly decreases the composite endpoint of hospitalization; thus, its use for persistent AF is becoming increasingly significant. Although persistent AF is associated with non-PV foci ectopy, degeneration of the atrial substrate also contributes greatly to persistent AF. To improve the outcomes of persistent AF, ablations other than PVI targeting the left atrial substrate published in recent reports are described below.

3.1 Complex fractionated atrial electrogram (CFAE)

Nademanee et al. defined local potentials (cycle length ≤ 120 ms) or continuously fractionated potentials as complex fractionated atrial electrogram (CFAE). According to Nademanee et al., CFAE during AF indicates regions of slow conduction and pivot points, within which ablation can terminate AF. However, CFAE does not always imply a reentry circuit that sustains AF; rather, it sometimes indicates the regions in which the excitable media that underlie fibrillation can be passively propagated or the etiology of AF is not connected. The Substrate and Trigger Ablation for Reduction of Atrial Fibrillation (STAR AF II) trial [16] demonstrated that CFAE showed no significant difference when compared with PVI alone in terms of prevention of AF recurrence. Therefore, this method has not been used in recent years.

3.2 Linear ablation

Linear ablation has been used previously. The most common linear ablations consist of a "roof line" that creates an ablation line connecting the right and left superior PVs and a "mitral isthmus line" creating an ablation line connecting the posterolateral mitral annulus and the left inferior PV. However, because the linear ablation technique is difficult to perform in many cases, prolonged procedure time and complications occasionally occur. Additionally, residual conduction gaps may cause recurrent arrhythmias.

In the STAR AF II trial, no significant difference was reported between linear ablation and PVI alone in terms of preventing AF recurrence.

3.3 Non-PV foci

Ablation of PVI and non-PV foci is necessary to improve treatment outcomes. Non-PV foci arise from the superior vena cava, left atrial posterior wall, atrial septum, mitral annulus, ligament of Marshall, coronary sinus, and crista terminalis. Active induction is often required to identify non-PV foci. When AF lasts longer, cardioversion is used to restore sinus rhythm. When AF recurs, it is necessary to identify its triggers. During sinus rhythm, induction is attempted by isoproterenol loading, ATP loading, and atrial pacing. To enable wide mapping, multiple electrodes are placed at various locations, and the region originating from the non-PV foci, which act as AF triggers, is identified from the early electric potentials recorded.

3.4 Ganglionated plexus

Ganglionated plexuses (GPs), which are mainly embedded within fat pads distributed to the epicardial surface of the atrium, contain the same number of cholinergic and adrenergic neurons. The cell bodies of GP neurons are densely populated by the following five areas of left atrial GPs: superior left GP, Marshall tract GP, anterior right GP, inferior left GP, and inferior right GP. GP ablation makes it possible to inhibit and eliminate both PV firing and fractionated atrial potential. According to Nakagawa et al. [17], among 63 patients with paroxysmal AF who underwent GP ablation and PVI, 90% did not experience AF recurrence at 1 year of follow-up.

3.5 CARTOFINDER™

The CARTOFINDER™ mapping system for AF catheter ablation, which was developed in recent years, enables the generation of wavefront propagation maps acquired from bipolar and unipolar signals using a 64-pole basket catheter. After filtering the ventricular activation signals, the unipolar signal created between two neighboring bipolar signals is annotated, and the focal and rotational activities are recorded. Ablation is performed on these drivers that terminates AF. The effectiveness of this ablation was reported previously, and future reports on clinical outcomes are expected.

3.6 ExTRa Mapping™

To completely cure patients with persistent AF using catheter ablation, it is necessary to determine the location of AF drivers in the atria. Ashihara et al. developed the first online real-time clinical arrhythmia visualization system, the ExTRa Mapping™.

This system includes specialized artificial intelligence based on intracardiac electrocardiography signals recorded by a 20-pole spiral-shaped catheter inserted into the atrium and visualizes arrhythmia by combining the action potential waveform of the human atrial muscle calculated by computer simulation. Highly intensified rotor sites in the visualized areas are ablated.

3.7 Low-voltage area ablation

This ablation procedure targets the low-voltage area in AF. However, it has limitations; for example, the definition of low-voltage areas is inconsistent, the low-voltage area can be influenced by map density or mapping catheter, and mapping during AF may overestimate the low-voltage area [18].

3.8 Left atrial appendage isolation

The left atrial appendage, a known frequent origin of non-PV triggers [19], is likely involved in the sustained form of AF. Left atrial appendage isolation carries the risk of cardiac perforation. Furthermore, patients who undergo isolation must be placed on lifelong anticoagulation therapy or undergo left atrial appendage closure; therefore, indications for this procedure must be carefully considered [20].

4. Predictive factors of AF recurrence after ablation

Advances in ablation techniques have improved the prognosis for paroxysmal AF. However, the prognosis remains inadequate. To identify patients with a good prognosis, it is necessary to use a new index.

4.1 AF duration

Our study [21] enrolled 82 consecutive patients (mean age, 65.0 ± 12.4 years), including 45 with persistent AF and 37 with long-standing persistent AF. The recurrence rate after ablation was high among patients with long-standing persistent AF. According to Watanabe et al. [22], compared with paroxysmal AF, persistent AF showed a higher recurrence rate after ablation but a lower rate of long-standing persistent AF. Generally, the longer the AF duration, the higher the AF recurrence rate.

4.2 Defibrillation threshold

We studied postprocedural ablation predictors of AF recurrence after univariate and multivariate analyses in 82 patients.10 J was considered the average DFT for persistent AF and set as the cutoff value, as a review article [23] reported that the average DFT for intracardiac cardioversion (IC) of 25 patients with persistent AF was 9.1 ± 7.4 J. In patients with persistent AF, the AF recurrence rate increased with DFT for IC despite the addition of radiofrequency applications after PVI (such as box isolation). We demonstrated that the high DFT was the strongest prognostic factor for AF recurrence after the ablation procedure. Therefore, we speculate that the high DFT is correlated with atrial remodeling, which gradually decreases the success rate of catheter ablation in AF.

4.3 Left atrial diameter, left atrial volume

Liu et al. reported that left atrial diameter (LAD) contributes to the prognosis of patients with AF after catheter ablation [24]. Moreover, Pinto et al. reported that left atrial appendage volume contributes to AF recurrence [25]. In contrast, Masuda et al. [26] reported that LAD and AF recurrence are not correlated; thus, whether they are related remains controversial. In contrast, a review article of a meta-analysis reported that left atrial volume is a predictor of atrial fibrillation recurrence [27].

4.4 Brain natriuretic peptide

Zyng et al. reported that high brain natriuretic peptide (BNP) levels were associated with AF recurrence after catheter ablation [28]. In contrast, we studied postprocedural ablation predictors of AF recurrence after univariate and multivariate analyses in 82 patients, which found no relationship between BNP level and AF recurrence. This might be attributed to the policy of the institute, in which AF ablation is performed after adequate medical treatment for heart failure is administered. Thus, the relationship between BNP level and AF recurrence after catheter ablation requires further investigation.

4.5 Ejection fraction

Our 82-patient study on postprocedural ablation predictors of AF recurrence demonstrated no correlation between ejection fraction (EF) and AF recurrence after ablation. Watanabe et al. reported similar results, indicating that EF is not a prognostic or predictive factor for AF recurrence after ablation.

4.6 Serum creatinine levels

Our 82-patient study on postprocedural ablation predictors of AF recurrence showed no correlation between serum creatinine levels and AF recurrence after ablation. Watanabe et al. similarly stated that creatinine clearance <50 mL/min was not a predictive factor for AF recurrence. Therefore, serum creatinine level is not a prognostic or predictive factor for AF recurrence.

5. Conclusion

Patients with paroxysmal AF who underwent PVI alone had a good prognosis, suggesting that ablation is an established treatment for paroxysmal AF. However, PVI alone for persistent AF may not prevent AF recurrence; thus, additional ablation approaches combined with PVI have been developed. No current procedure clearly shows a preventive effect on AF recurrence; therefore, this issue remains controversial. To improve treatment outcomes of the ablation of persistent AF, it is necessary to identify patients who are most likely to experience the maximum therapeutic effect. Therefore, AF duration and DFT and left atrial volume could be indicators. Future large-scale studies are necessary.

Acknowledgements

The author thanks EDITAGE for providing English language editing.

Conflict of interest

The author declares no conflicts of interest.

Author details

Kohei Sawasaki
Department of Cardiology, Hamamatsu Medical Center, Hamamatsu, Shizuoka, Japan

*Address all correspondence to: sawasaki@hmedc.or.jp

References

[1] Wyse DG, Waldo AL, DiMarco JP, et al. A comparison of rate control and rhythm control in patients with atrial fibrillation. The New England Journal of Medicine. 2002;**347**:1825-1833

[2] Haïssaguerre M, Jaïs P, Shah DC, et al. Spontaneous initiation of atrial fibrillation by ectopic beats originating in the pulmonary veins. The New England Journal of Medicine. 1998;**339**:659-666

[3] Packer DL, Mark DB, Robb RA, et al. Effect of catheter ablation vs antiarrhythmic drug therapy on mortality, stroke, bleeding, and cardiac arrest among patients with atrial fibrillation: The CABANA randomized clinical trial. Journal of the American Medical Association. 2019;**321**(13):1261-1274

[4] Marrouche NF, Brachmann J, Andresen D, et al. Catheter ablation for atrial fibrillation with heart failure. The New England Journal of Medicine. 2018;**378**:417-427

[5] Kuck K-H, Brugada J, Fürnkranz A, et al. Cryoballoon or radiofrequency ablation for paroxysmal atrial fibrillation. The New England Journal of Medicine. 2016;**374**:2235-2245

[6] Yamane T. Catheter ablation of atrial fibrillation. Medical View. 2009:86-94

[7] Nademanee K, McKenzie J, Kosar E, et al. A new approach for catheter ablation of atrial fibrillation: Mapping of the electrophysiologic substrate. Journal of the American College of Cardiology. 2004;**43**(11):2044-2053

[8] Honarbakhsh S, Schilling RJ, Dhillon G, et al. A novel mapping system for panoramic mapping of the left atrium: Application to detect and characterize localized sources maintaining atrial fibrillation. JACC: Clinical Electrophysiology. 2018;**4**(1):124-134

[9] Ashihara T. Catheter ablation based on real-time visualization of non-paroxismal atrial fibrillation. Igakunoayumi. 2020;(6):733-740

[10] Fukamizu S. Keys to successful catheter ablation. Medical View. 2018:190-199

[11] Kokubo Y, Matsumoto C. Traditional cardiovascular risk factors for incident atrial fibrillation. Circulation Journal. 2016;**80**:2415-2422

[12] Lin Y, Chen Y, Lee T, Chen Y, Chen S, Chen Y. Aging modulates the substrate and triggers remodeling in atrial fibrillation. Circulation Journal. 2018;**82**:1237-1244

[13] Dukkipati SR, Cuoco F, Kutinsky I, et al. Pulmonary vein isolation using the visually guided laser balloon: A prospective, multicenter, and randomized comparison to standard radiofrequency ablation. Journal of the American College of Cardiology. 2015;**66**(12):1350-1360

[14] Satake S. Hot balloon catheter ablation of atrial fibrillation. Kinpodo. 2017:13-20

[15] Goya M. Features of ablation catheter and how to use them. Heartview. 2022;**26**(2):51-55

[16] Verma A, Jiang C, Betts TR, et al. Approaches to catheter ablation for persistent atrial fibrillation. The New England Journal of Medicine. 2015;**372**:1812-1822

[17] Nakagawa H. Practical Approach to Catheter Ablation of Atrial Fibrillation. Philadelphia: Lippincott Williams & Wilkins; 2008. pp. 218-230

[18] Yamashita S. Visually guided laser ablation and catheter ablation for press latest atrial fibrillation. Igakunoayumi. 2019;(4):249-256

[19] Di Biase L, Burkhardt JD, Mohanty P, et al. Left atrial appendage: An underrecognized trigger site of atrial fibrillation. Circulation. 2010;**122**(2):109-118

[20] Nishimura M, Lupercio-Lopez F, Hsu JC. Left atrial appendage electrical isolation as a target in atrial fibrillation. JACC: Clinical Electrophysiology. 2019;**5**(4):407-416

[21] Sawasaki K, Inden Y, Hosoya N, et al. Defibrillation threshold of internal cardioversion prior to ablation predicts atrial fibrillation recurrence. Clinical Cardiology. 2021;**44**(8):1169-1176

[22] Watanabe R, Nagashima K, Wakamatsu Y, et al. Different determinants of the recurrence of atrial fibrillation and adverse clinical events in the mid-term period after atrial fibrillation ablation. Circulation Journal. 2022;**86**(2):233-242

[23] Boriani G, Biffi M, Camanini C, Luceri RM, Branzi A. Transvenous low energy internal cardioversion for atrial fibrillation: A review of clinical applications and future developments. PACE. 2001;**24**:99-107

[24] Liu J, Yang H, Liu Y, et al. Early recurrence of atrial tachyarrhythmia during the 90-day blanking period after cryoballoon ablation in patients with atrial fibrillation: the characteristics and predictive value of early recurrence on long-term outcomes. Journal of Electrocardiology. 2020;**58**:46-50

[25] Teixeira PP, Oliveira MM, Ramos R, et al. Left atrial appendage volume as a new predictor of atrial fibrillation recurrence after catheter ablation. Journal of Interventional Cardiac Electrophysiology. 2017;**49**:165-171

[26] Masuda M, Fujita M, Iida O, et al. Left atrial low-voltage area predict atrial defibrillation recurrence after catheter ablation in patients with paroxysmal atrial fibrillation. International Journal of Cardiology. 2018;**257**:97-101

[27] Njoku A, Kannabhiran M, Arora R, et al. Left atrial volume predicts atrial fibrillation recurrence after radiofrequency ablation: A meta-analysis. Europace. 2018;**20**(1):33-42

[28] Zhang Y, Chen A, Song L, Li M, Chen Y, He B. Association between baseline natriuretic peptides and atrial fibrillation recurrence after catheter ablation. A meta-analysis. International Heart Journal. 2016;**57**:183-189

Chapter 3

Advances in the Nonpharmacological Treatment of Atrial Fibrillation

Manuel Lorenzo López Reboiro, Raul Franco Gutierrez, Laura Ramos Rúa, María del Carmen Basalo Carbajales, Laura Rodrigo Lara, Candela Fraga González, Celia Sobrado Moreiras, José Manuel Cerqueiro González and José López Castro

Abstract

Atrial fibrillation is a very frequent arrhythmia in our daily clinical practice, either isolated or associated with other heart diseases. It has high relevance as it can act as a decompensating agent of other heart diseases or damage the myocardium itself. Traditionally, the treatment of atrial fibrillation has been based on rhythm and rate control and also the treatment of its complications. To rhythm control, electrical or pharmacological cardioversion has been used, and different groups of brady-cardizing drugs have been used for rate control. Anticoagulation is the most relevant treatment to prevent thromboembolic phenomena secondary to atrial fibrillation. However, with the recent development of endovascular procedures, the use of ablation to maintain sinus rhythm in this kind of patients has been increased displacing the use of other treatment strategies. Therefore, in this chapter, we would review the present evidence in the use of ablation techniques as atrial fibrillation treatment.

Keywords: atrial fibrillation, ablation, rhythm control

1. Introduction

Atrial fibrillation is the most frequent sustained cardiac arrhythmia in adults. It has two differential characteristics, one electrocardiographic and another clinical.

Clinically it is characterized by an irregularly irregular pulse, due to a supraventricular tachycardia producing a chaotic atrial activity. In addition, the electrocardiogram (ECG) shows the following defining characteristics [1]:

- Irregular R-R interval

- Absence of P waves
- Irregular atrial activation (f waves)

Nowadays, the prevalence of this arrhythmia is rising due to, among to other causes, the increase in life expectancy and the effort to diagnose it [2]. In addition to the importance of this fact, AF has a special relevance resulting from its treatments and its complications, existing multiple pharmacologic treatments to control the harmful effects of this arrhythmia on patients. However, there are alternatives to pharmacological treatments that we would like to summarize in this chapter.

1.1 Types of AF

To be considered as AF, the arrhythmia must be documented by ECG and lasts >30 seconds [3]. If these two features are met, the arrhythmia is called clinical AF, and if not, the arrhythmia is considered as an rapid atrial rate episode or subclinical AF.

Based on the time of evolution, the AF is classified as [4]:

- First diagnosed AF: AF has not been diagnosed before.
- Paroxysmal AF: self-terminated or cardioverted within 7 days.
- Persistent AF: AF that lasts longer than 7 days, but it is still considered rhythm control strategy.
- Permanent AF: Rate control but not rhythm control is pursued.

1.2 Predisposing factor for AF

There are a number of factors that predispose to AF, including [5–7]:

- Older age
- High blood pressure
- Type 2 diabetes mellitus
- Heart failure
- Coronary disease
- Chronic kidney disease
- Obesity
- Obstructive sleep apnea

These risk factors contribute to the damage in the atrial as changes in the structure, architecture, contractility, and electrophysiology that may lead to the dilatation, fibrosis, dysfunction, and distortion conduction in the left atrial. This cumulative damage is the substrate on which atrial fibrillation develops [8].

2. Diagnosis

Diagnosis of AF requires rhythm documentation on an ECG showing this arrhythmia lasting at least 30 seconds. There are other ways to detect AF that will require further diagnostic confirmation by performing a 12-lead ECG and interpretation by an experienced physician.

There are multiple tools that can be used to screen for atrial fibrillation:

- Blood pressure monitor
- Pulse palpation
- ECG Holter monitor
- Single-lead ECG
- Implanted cardiac devices
- Hospital telemetry/noninvasive long-term ECG monitoring
- Smartwatches
- Mobile devices

Most recently, mobile devices are increasingly being used as screening tools as they are becoming easy to use and are widely distributed among the population.

These devices perform the interpretation of the electrical tracing through applications. Currently there are studies carried out by the different companies that manufacture mobile devices. (e.g., Estudio Apple Heart) [9, 10].

The opportunistic AF screening with these devices is cost-effective, but the diagnostic efforts must be done in those high-risk patients, who are those older than 65 years and at risk of stroke [9, 11].

3. Treatment

AF treatment is fundamentally based on rhythm and heart rate control and its thrombotic complications. Lately, multiple drugs and therapeutic attitudes have been developed for this purpose. In this section, we will show a few hints about nonpharmacological treatments for atrial fibrillation, often less known and used than conventional treatments, which are much more widespread.

3.1 Cardioembolic events prevention

AF increases the risk of cardioembolic events. There are several scales to quantify this risk, and the most widely used is the CHA2DS2-VASC scale. Only the patients with low risk would not need to take preventive treatment [12].

Anticoagulant treatments are the most known choice to prevent cardioembolic events secondary to AF. These include vitamin-K-dependent (AVK) and nondependent (NAVK) anticoagulants. However, there is a nonpharmacological alternative for stroke prevention, the surgical left atrial appendage occlusion (LAAO) or exclusion. This technique has shown to be noninferior to VKA anticoagulation for stroke prevention in patients with AF and moderate risk of stroke [13].

This technique is reserved for patients with absolute contraindications to pharmacological anticoagulation. The contraindications are as follows [14]:

- Severe active bleeding
- Severe thrombocytopenia
- Severe anemia
- Very high risk of bleeding risk

There are two main techniques to LAA occlusion/exclusion, either by devices or by cardiac surgery. The last one is left as an alternative when invasive treatment is to be performed, such as cardiac surgery for another cause or when surgical ablation of AF is performed [15].

These techniques has the advantage that they will not require subsequent anticoagulation, so they are exempt from the hemorrhagic complications derived from anticoagulant treatment maintained over time. On the other hand, these patients will need antiplatelet treatment for life [16].

3.2 Rate control therapy in atrial fibrillation

This is one of the mainstay established in the AF control. As the name suggests, this measure aims to control the patient's heart rate without attempting to restore sinus rhythm, allowing AF to remain.

However, there is a serious controversy among the targets set out because to date it has not been established which attitude is more favorable for the patient, strict heart rate (HR) control <80 bpm, or a more permissive one <110 bpm [17]. Nevertheless, there is certainty that the heart rate should be controlled at the acute moment when it produces hemodynamic instability as quickly as possible and with fewer side effects for the patient.

Pharmacological treatments are the first-line treatments, and there is a wide range of therapeutic families from which to choose the best alternative. When pharmacological treatment fails, there is another alternative, such as atrioventricular node ablation and subsequent implantation of a pacemaker [18]. The efficacy of the procedure improves when the pacemaker is implanted a few weeks before the AV nodal ablation, and the initial pacing rate after ablation is set at 70–90 bpm [19].

Within this technique there are variants because in patients with permanent AF hospitalized due to heart failure, it can be considered the implantation of resynchronization devices or even the His bundle pacing [19, 20].

3.3 Rhythm control therapy in atrial fibrillation

This is the last mainstay we will deal with in this review. As in the previous section, there are several pharmacological treatments approved for this purpose, but we also have available nonpharmacological treatments with proved efficacy.

The fundamental purpose to rhythm control is to reduce symptoms related to AF and improve patients' quality of life. In addition, it reduces the AF progression rate and the deleterious anatomopathological changes caused by AF on the myocardium [21, 22].

Among the nonpharmacological options to try to keep patients in sinus rhythm, we would like to outline the electrical cardioversion, AF ablation, and AF surgery.

3.3.1 Electrical cardioversion

This technique has the advantage of allowing immediate cardioversion, which makes it the technique of choice in patients with hemodynamically unstable AF, although it is also used for elective cardioversion. It is faster and more effective than pharmacological cardioversion [23, 24].

Electrical cardioversion is performed with directly and synchronous biphasic defibrillators with maximum power and placing the electrodes in an anteroposterior position [23, 25].

This is a painful procedure, and it is not exempt from complications. For this reason, the patient must be properly sedated and monitored in order to be able to handle any incidents that may arise [26].

This is a very effective technique, but there are factors that increase the risk of recurrence after cardioversion [27]:

- Older age
- Female sex
- Previous failed cardioversion
- Chronic obstructive pulmonary disease
- Renal failure
- Structural cardiopathy
- Heart failure
- Dilated left atria

3.3.2 Catheter ablation of AF

Catheter ablation is a recognized technique for preventing AF recurrence, but there are several factors that increase the risk of failure [28, 29]:

- Older age
- Renal disease
- Left atrial size
- AF duration

- AF substrate in an MRI study
- Intensive control of AF risk factors could decrease the AF recurrence rate after ablation [30].

The aim of ablation is to improve patients' symptoms and quality of life, as it has not demonstrated in general population to reduce neither patients' mortality nor preventing cardioembolic events or bleedings related to pharmacologic treatment [31]. However, it has shown benefits in selected population as they are patients with heart failure and depressed ventricular ejection fraction and also when AF-mediated tachycardia induced cardiomyopathy is suspected, because in these cases can improve the left ventricular function [31, 32].

Therefore, the indications for catheter ablation of AF are as follows:

- Second-line treatment after anti-arrhythmic medications
- Paroxysmal or recurrent AF in patients without recurrence risk factors

Ablation versus pharmacological treatment as first-line treatment of paroxysmal AF has shown to have a lower recurrent atrial arrhythmias rate, similar risk of serious adverse events, and lower consumption of healthcare resources [33].

The technique consists of the complete electrical pulmonary veins isolation by sequential ablation with radiofrequency or cryoablation around the atrioventricular junction or with single-discharge devices, although electrical isolation is very difficult, so if the point of origin of the arrhythmia is not detected, more extensive ablations tend to be performed [34, 35]. The procedure is not exempted of complications, even though they are unfrequent: periprocedure death, esophageal perforation, thromboembolism, cardiac tamponade, pulmonary veins stenosis, phrenic nerve permanent paralysis... [36].

3.3.3 AF surgery

The technique of choice is the COX procedure, which, like ablation, has an impact on patients' quality of life, but not on the other indicators [37]. Recurrence risk factors are also overlappable to those of AF catheter ablation.

AF surgery is usually performed in the context of other cardiac surgery, such as mitral valve repair, but can also be performed in isolation demonstrating less need for repeat procedure than in cases where ablation was performed, but with longer hospital stays and more frequent complications [38, 39].

Surgery can also be concomitantly performed with ablation, improving the results respect to both techniques separately, but having more complications than when ablation is done alone [24].

4. Summary of AF treatments

- Thrombotic events prevention:

  a. Left atrial appendage occlusion or exclusion: recommended in patients with contraindications to anticoagulation therapies.

- Rate control:

    a. Atrioventricular node ablation and subsequent implantation of a pacemaker: recommended in selected patients when pharmacologic treatment is ineffective or contraindicated.

    b. Rhythm control:

        i. Electric cardioversion:

            1. Urgent: performed in patients with hemodynamic instability

            2. Elective: performed in patients in whom pharmacological treatment has failed

        ii. Catheter ablation:

            1. Second-line therapy after pharmacologic treatment

            2. First-line treatment in selected patients

        iii. AF surgery: recommended in patients who are already undergoing cardiac surgery for another reason. For example, mitral valve prosthetic replacement.

        iv. Hybrid technique of AF surgery and ablation: recommended for refractory cases.

5. Conclusion

After this review, we can conclude that the procedures of choice for the treatment of atrial fibrillation are the less invasive, so the fundamental pillar remains pharmacological treatments. However, there are a number of alternatives that can be used when pharmacological treatments fail, when they are contraindicated or in electively, so we have to keep them in mind to enrich our therapeutic arsenal. Moreover, these techniques are a safe and effective solution and are widely supported by the literature.

Conflict of interest

The authors declare no conflict of interest.

Author details

Manuel Lorenzo López Reboiro[1*], Raul Franco Gutierrez[2], Laura Ramos Rúa[3], María del Carmen Basalo Carbajales[4], Laura Rodrigo Lara[5], Candela Fraga González[1], Celia Sobrado Moreiras[1], José Manuel Cerqueiro González[6] and José López Castro[1]

1 Internal Medicine Department, Public Hospital Monforte de Lemos, Lugo, Spain

2 Cardiology Department, University Hospital Lucus Augusti, Lugo, Spain

3 Neurology Department, University Hospital Lucus Augusti, Lugo, Spain

4 Cardiology Department, University Hospital Bellvitge, L'Hospitalet de Llobregat, Barcelona, Spain

5 Internal Medicine Department, University Hospital Ourense, Ourense, Spain

6 Internal Medicine Department, University Hospital Lucus Augusti, Lugo, Spain

*Address all correspondence to: manuel.lorenzo.lopez.reboiro@sergas.es

References

[1] Hindricks G, Potpara T, Dagres N, et al. Guia ESC 2020sobre el diagnóstico y tratamiento de la fibrilación auricular, desarrollada en colaboración dela European Association for Cardio-Thoracic Surgery (EACTS). Revista Española de Cardiología. 2021;**74**(5):437e1-437e1. DOI: 10.1016/j.recesp.2000.1.017

[2] Ren J, Pan G, Yang J, et al. Circ_0000620 acts as an oncogenic factor in gastric cancer through regulating MMP2 expression via sponging miR-671-5p. Journal of Biological Research (Thessalon). 2021;**28**(1):23. DOI: 10.1186/s40709-021-00154-5

[3] Verma A, Boersma L, Haines DE, et al. First-in-Human Experience and Acute Procedural Outcomes Using a Novel Pulsed Field Ablation System: The PULSED AF Pilot Trial. Circulation: Arrhythmia and Electrophysiology. 2022;**15**(1):e010168. DOI: 10.1161/CIRCEP.121.010168

[4] Kirchhof P, Benussi S, Kotecha D, et al. ESC Scientific Document Group. 2016 ESC Guidelines for the management of atrial fibrillation developed in collaboration with EACTS. European Heart Journal. 2016;**37**(38):2893-2962. DOI: 10.1093/eurheartj/ehw210

[5] Boriani G, Savelieva I, Dan GA, et al. Document reviewers. Chronic kidney disease in patients with cardiac rhythm disturbances or implantable electrical devices: Clinical significance and implications for decision making-a position paper of the European Heart Rhythm Association endorsed by the Heart Rhythm Society and the Asia Pacific Heart Rhythm Society. Europace. 2015;**17**(8):1169-1196. DOI: 10.1093/europace/euv202

[6] Aune D, Feng T, Schlesinger S, et al. Diabetes mellitus, blood glucose and the risk of atrial fibrillation: A systematic review and meta-analysis of cohort studies. Journal of Diabetes and its Complications. 2018;**32**(5):501-511. DOI: 10.1016/j.jdiacomp.2018.02.004

[7] Lip GYH, Coca A, Kahan T, et al. Hypertension and cardiac arrhythmias: A consensus document from the European Heart Rhythm Association (EHRA) and ESC Council on Hypertension, endorsed by the Heart Rhythm Society (HRS), Asia-Pacific Heart Rhythm Society (APHRS) and Sociedad Latinoamericana de Estimulación Cardíaca y Electrofisiología (SOLEACE). Europace. 2017;**19**(6):891-911. DOI: 10.1093/europace/eux091

[8] Goette A, Kalman JM, Aguinaga L, et al. Document reviewers: EHRA/HRS/APHRS/SOLAECE expert consensus on atrial cardiomyopathies: Definition, characterization, and clinical implication. Europace. 2016;**18**(10):1455-1490. DOI: 10.1093/europace/euw161

[9] Mairesse GH, Moran P, Van Gelder IC, et al. ESC Scientific Document Group. Screening for atrialfibrillation: A European Heart Rhythm Association (EHRA) consensus documentendorsed by the Heart Rhythm Society (HRS) Asia Pacific Heart Rhythm Society(APHRS), and Sociedad Latinoamericana de Estimulación Cardiaca yElectrofisiología (SOLAECE). Europace. 2017;**19**:1589-1623

[10] Schnabel RB, Haeusler KG, Healey JS, et al. Searching for atrial fibrillation poststroke: A white paper of the AF-SCREEN international collaboration. Circulation.

2019;**140**(22):1834-1850. DOI: 10.1161/CIRCULATIONAHA.119.040267

[11] Hobbs FD, Fitzmaurice DA, Mant J, et al. A randomised controlled trial and cost-effectiveness study ofsystematic screening (targeted and total population screening) versus routinepractice for the detection of atrial fibrillation in people aged 65 and over TheSAFE study. Health Technology Assessment. 2005;**9**:1-74

[12] Lip GY, Nieuwlaat R, Pisters R, et al. Refining clinical risk stratificationfor predicting Stroke and thromboembolism in atrial fibrillation using anovel risk factor-based approach: The Euro Heart Survey on atrial fibrillation. Chest. 2010;**137**:263-272

[13] Holmes DR, Doshi SK, Kar S, et al. Left atrial appendage closure as an alternative to warfarin forStroke prevention in atrial fibrillation: A patient-level meta-analysis. Journal of American College of Cardiology. 2015;**65**:2614-2623

[14] Boersma LV, Ince H, Kische S, et al. EWOLUTION Investigators. Efficacy and safety of left atrial appendage closure with WATCHMAN in patients with or without contraindication to oral anticoagulation: 1-Year follow-up outcome data of the EWOLUTION trial. Heart Rhythm. 2017 Sep;**14**(9):1302-1308

[15] Tsai YC, Phan K, Munkholm-Larsen S, et al. Surgical left atrial appendage occlusion during cardiac surgery for patients with atrial fibrillation: A meta-analysis. European Journal of Cardio-Thoracic Surgery. 2015;**47**(5):847-854. DOI: 10.1093/ejcts/ezu291

[16] Tilz RR, Potpara T, Chen J, et al. Left atrial appendage occluder implantation in Europe: Indications and anticoagulation post-implantation. Results of the European Heart Rhythm Association Survey. Europace. 2017;**19**(10):1737-1742. DOI: 10.1093/europace/eux254

[17] Groenveld HF, Crijns HJ, Van den Berg MP, et al. The effect of rate control on quality of life in patients with permanent atrial fibrillation: Data from the RACE II (Rate Control Efficacy in Permanent Atrial Fibrillation II) study. Journal of the American College of Cardiology. 2011;**58**(17):1795-1803. DOI: 10.1016/j.jacc.2011.06.055

[18] Lim KT, Davis MJ, Powell A, et al. Ablate and pace strategy for atrial fibrillation: Long-term outcome of AIRCRAFT trial. Europace. 2007;**9**(7):498-505. DOI: 10.1093/europace/eum091

[19] Wang RX, Lee HC, Hodge DO, et al. Effect of pacing method on risk of sudden death after atrioventricular node ablation and pacemaker implantation in patients with atrial fibrillation. Heart Rhythm. 2013;**10**(5):696-701. DOI: 10.1016/j.hrthm.2013.01.021

[20] Huang W, Su L, Wu S, et al. Benefits of Permanent his bundle pacing combined with atrioventricular node ablation in atrial fibrillation patients with heart failure with both preserved and reduced left ventricular ejection fraction. Journal of the American Heart Association 2017 Apr 1;**6**(4):e005309

[21] Bunch TJ, May HT, Bair TL, et al. Increasing time between first diagnosis of atrial fibrillation and catheter ablation adversely affects long-term outcomes. Heart Rhythm. 2013;**10**(9):1257-1262. DOI: 10.1016/j.hrthm.2013.05.013

[22] Teh AW, Kistler PM, Lee G, Medi C, et al. Long-term effects of catheter ablation for lone atrial fibrillation:

Progressive atrial electroanatomic substrate remodeling despite successful ablation. Heart Rhythm. 2012;**9**(4):473-480. DOI: 10.1016/j.hrthm.2011.11.013

[23] Kirchhof P, Mönnig G, Wasmer K, et al. A trial of self-adhesive patch electrodes and hand-held paddle electrodes for external cardioversion of atrial fibrillation (MOBIPAPA). European Heart Journal. 2005;**26**(13):1292-1297. DOI: 10.1093/eurheartj/ehi160

[24] Soulat-Dufour L, Lang S, Addetia K, et al. Restoring sinus rhythm reverses cardiac remodeling and reduces valvular regurgitation in patients with atrial fibrillation. Journal of the American College of Cardiology. 2022;**79**(10):951-961. DOI: 10.1016/j.jacc.2021.12.029

[25] Inácio JF et al. Monophasic and biphasic shock for transthoracic conversion of atrial fibrillation: Systematic review and network meta-analysis. Resuscitation. 2016;**100**:66-75. DOI: 10.1016/j.resuscitation.2015.12.009

[26] Furniss SS, Sneyd JR. Safe sedation in modern cardiological practice. Heart. 2015;**101**(19):1526-1530. DOI: 10.1136/heartjnl-2015-307656

[27] Toufan M, Kazemi B, Molazadeh N. The significance of the left atrial volume index in prediction of atrial fibrillation recurrence after electrical cardioversion. Journal of Cardiovascular and Thoracic Research. 2017;**9**(1):54-59. DOI: 10.15171/jcvtr.2017.08

[28] Marrouche NF, Wilber D, Hindricks G, et al. Association of atrial tissue fibrosis identified by delayed enhancement MRI and atrial fibrillation catheter ablation: The DECAAF study. Journal of the American Medical Association. 2014;**311**(5):498-506. DOI: 10.1001/jama.2014.3

[29] Li Z, Wang S, Hidru TH, et al. Fibrillation duration and early recurrence are reliable predictors of late recurrence after radiofrequency catheter ablation. Frontiers in Cardiovascular Medicine. 2022;**9**:864417. DOI: 10.3389/fcvm.2022.864417

[30] Pathak RK, Middeldorp ME, Lau DH, et al. Aggressive risk factor reduction study for atrial fibrillation and implications for the outcome of ablation: The ARREST-AF cohort study. Journal of the American College of Cardiology. 2014;**64**(21):2222-2231. DOI: 10.1016/j.jacc.2014.09.028

[31] Reddy VY, Dukkipati SR, Neuzil P, et al. Randomized, controlled trial of the safety and effectiveness of a contact force-sensing irrigated catheter for ablation of paroxysmal atrial fibrillation: Results of the tacticath contact force ablation catheter study for atrial fibrillation (TOCCASTAR) study. Circulation. 2015;**132**(10):907-915. DOI: 10.1161/CIRCULATIONAHA.114.014092

[32] Hindricks G, Sepehri Shamloo A, Lenarczyk R, et al. Catheter ablation of atrial fibrillation: Current status, techniques, outcomes and challenges. Kardiologia Polska. 2018;**76**(12):1680-1686. DOI: 10.5603/KP.a2018.0216

[33] Imberti JF, Ding WY, Kotalczyk A, et al. Catheter ablation as first-line treatment for paroxysmal atrial fibrillation: A systematic review and meta-analysis. Heart. 2021;**107**(20):1630-1636. DOI: 10.1136/heartjnl-2021-319496

[34] Kircher S, Arya A, Altmann D, Rolf S, et al. Individually tailored vs. standardized substrate modification duringradiofrequency catheter ablation for atrial fibrillation: A randomized study. Europace. 2018;**20**:1766-1775

[35] Arbelo E, Brugada J, Blomström-Lundqvist C, et al. On the behalf of the ESC-EHRA Atrial Fibrillation Ablation Long-term Registry Investigators. Contemporary management of patients undergoing atrial fibrillation ablation: In-hospital and 1-year follow-up findings from the ESC-EHRA atrial fibrillation ablation long-term registry. European Heart Journal. 2017;**38**(17):1303-1316. DOI: 10.1093/eurheartj/ehw564

[36] Bagge L, Probst J, Jensen SM, et al. Quality of life is not improved after mitral valve surgery combined with epicardial left atrial cryoablation as compared with mitral valve surgery alone: A substudy of the double blind randomized SWEDish Multicentre Atrial Fibrillation study (SWEDMAF). Europace. 2018;**20**(FI_3):f343-f350. DOI: 10.1093/europace/eux253

[37] Kim HJ, Kim JS, Kim TS. Epicardial thoracoscopic ablation versus endocardial catheter ablation for management of atrial fibrillation: A systematic review and meta-analysis. Interactive Cardiovascular and Thoracic Surgery. 2016;**22**:729-737

[38] Gammie JS, Haddad M, Milford-Beland S, et al. Atrial fibrillation correction surgery: Lessons from the Society of Thoracic Surgeons National Cardiac Database. The Annals of Thoracic Surgery. 2008;**85**:909-914

[39] van der Heijden CAJ, Vroomen M, Luermans JG, et al. Hybrid versus catheter ablation in patients with persistent and longstanding persistent atrial fibrillation: A systematic review and meta-analysis†. European Journal of Cardio-Thoracic Surgery. 2019;**56**(3):433-443. DOI: 10.1093/ejcts/ezy475

Chapter 4

Cardiovascular Magnetic Resonance Imaging of Atrial Fibrillation: An Advanced Hemodynamic Perspective

Mankarman Ghuman, Hansuk Kim, Hana Sheitt and Julio Garcia

Abstract

Atrial fibrillation (AF) patients can be referred to cardiac magnetic resonance imaging (MRI) for an accurate assessment of cardiac function and left atrial structure. Cardiac MRI is the gold standard for the quantification of heart volumes and allows the noninvasive tissue characterization of the heart. In addition, advanced flow assessment can be achieved using 4D-flow MRI to elegantly depict the hemodynamic efficiency of the left atrium (LA) and left ventricle (LV) throughout the cardiac cycle. Patients with AF may have occult LV disease and thrombus formation. Biomarkers based on 4D-flow MRI may unmask the presence of LA/LV disease by quantifying 3D stasis, flow distribution, and vortex formation. These biomarkers have proved to characterize AF stages, to complement standard risk scores, and bring new insights on heart hemodynamic performance. This chapter aims to present a standard cardiac MRI protocol for atrial fibrillation and the innovative usefulness of advanced flow imaging in clinical settings.

Keywords: cardiac flow, atrial fibrillation, 4D-flow magnetic resonance imaging (MRI), hemodynamic biomarkers

1. Introduction

Imaging and quantifying various characteristics of blood flow throughout the heart is essential in modern-day cardiology. Accurate image representations help accurately identify many known types of cardiovascular diseases. Atrial fibrillation (AF) is one of the most common types of atrial arrhythmias encountered in adults, which can be characterized by an irregular and rapid heartbeat with uncoordinated atrial activation and ineffective atrial contraction [1, 2]. The Framingham Heart Study reported that AF developed in 37% of the population after the age of 55 years [3]. AF can be detected and/or confirmed through various image modalities since it originates in the atrial chambers of the heart. This arrhythmia causes multiple simultaneous electrical signals firing within the atria leading to irregular electrocardiogram (ECG) patterns and atrial activity, loss of coordinated atrial contractions, and inadequate ventricular filling [4]. A patient with AF may experience symptoms, the most common of which include palpitations, shortness of breath, fatigue, dizziness, and chest pain [4].

AF can be caused by various factors. Individuals with previously existing cardiovascular diseases show higher signs of developing AF [4]. A common cause can be atrioventricular (AV) dyssynchrony, in which the normal AV contraction experiences delays due to the irregular conduction of the AV node [5]. AV dyssynchrony can be the reason behind the more common symptoms of AF since it directly affects the atria, causing it to operate in a fast and disorganized matter. There is a small fraction of patients who do not have previously existing heart problems yet still show signs of AF [4]. For these patients, AF can be a result of lifestyle choices, such as diet, lack of exercise, and smoking [6]. A recent multi-institutional study reported that 19% of patients newly diagnosed with AF (41% women) had an acute AF precipitant including mainly cardiac surgery (22%) and pneumonia (20%) followed in minor portion by myocardial infarction, pulmonary embolism, thyrotoxicosis, or alcohol intoxication [7].

A common mechanism for developing AF involves thrombogenicity. An increase in thrombogenicity within the heart can be a result of AF or can further increase the incidence of AF in patients who do not yet have it [8]. Intracardiac thrombi can be found in the atrial walls among patients with AF since the fast and irregular contractions of the atria can cause stress on the endometrial walls, resulting in damage, which promotes a hemostatic pathway to induce thrombus formation [9]. Another mechanism in AF involves hemodynamics. Specifically, decreased left ventricular (LV) hemodynamics can be affiliated with AF [10]. Maintaining adequate blood flow is important for overall cardiovascular health. Patients with AF typically show decreased hemodynamics; their low cardiac output can be attributed to irregular atrial contractions, causing their blood to begin pooling in the atria.

Mechanisms like increased thrombogenicity and decreased LV hemodynamics in patients with AF can lead to manifestations like stroke and ischemia. Increased thrombogenicity in the heart could cause a decrease in blood flow to the brain, resulting in a stroke [11]. A stroke would be a severe outcome as it drastically reduces overall body function and ability. Individuals with AF are much more likely to have a stroke in their lifetime than others since they have repeated incidents of irregular heartbeat [11]. This key symptom is what drives the formation of thrombi and can obstruct cardiac output. AF is associated with an increased incidence of stroke by a factor of four in men and 5.7 in women [12]. The risk of death increases by a factor of 2.4 among men and by a factor of 3.5 among women [13]. Reduced left atrium (LA) function increases the risk of blood stasis and clot formation in the LA, especially the left atrial appendage (LAA), which is a small extension of the LA. The LAA structure has high anatomical variability and has an important endocrine function. Its separation from the LA body promotes a blood turnover dependent on the systolic contraction. The loss of the LAA contraction during AF contributes to the increment of blood stasis and thrombus formation [14]. The CHA_2DS_2-VASc score considers the patient's history of congestive heart failure, hypertension, diabetes mellitus, stroke, vascular disease, age (between 65 and 74 years and >75 years), and sex. It is currently used for the stroke risk stratification of AF patients and for the recommendation of anticoagulant therapy [1, 2, 15]. However, the CHA_2DS_2-VASc score does not include individual physiologic factors, which limit its prediction power.

Another manifestation, ischemia, can be a result of decreased LV hemodynamics. Ischemia is a condition observed when there is an obstruction of blood flow to a part of the body or organ. An ischemic stroke, a combination of the two manifestations, could also be a possibility for individuals with AF as an obstruction in the circulatory system slows down cardiac output and causes low oxygen levels [16]. AF directly influences decreased cardiac output and can, therefore, be a leading factor in ischemic strokes seen in patients [1, 2]. At an early stage, an AF episode lasts <7 days of onset, and then, sinus rhythm is restored. This stage is known as paroxysmal AF. As severity progresses, AF episodes can last beyond 1 week. This stage is known as persistent AF. If the event does not terminate, it is considered as permanent AF. Persistent AF continues unless it is interrupted by electrical or pharmacological cardioversion, and it is associated with increased atrial fibrosis than paroxysmal AF [17]. Among patients undergoing cardioversion, up to 20% develop recurrent AF, and it becomes difficult to restore sinus rhythm [18].

There are many types of image modalities used to accurately diagnose several types of cardiovascular diseases. AF in patients can be identified using dedicated technology like electrocardiogram (ECG), echocardiogram (echo), cardiac computed tomography (CT), and cardiac magnetic resonance imaging (MRI). ECG is the best tool for recording electrical signals in the heart that correspond to the contraction and relaxation of the atria and ventricles. By performing ECG tests over long periods of time, a physician can recognize if there are any atrial arrhythmias like AF present by assessing the electrical patterns corresponding to the patient's heartbeat [19]. In patients that do not display visible signs of arrhythmias, yet present with symptoms, a Holter monitor can be used to assess any irregular heartbeats the patient may experience in a 24-hour period [20]. In addition to an echo and ECG, a CT scan can be used for detecting AF in patients. Unlike an ECG, a cardiac CT is a scan of the heart that shows any calcium deposits in the coronary arteries and chambers of the heart. Used mainly on patients presenting with symptoms of coronary heart disease, a CT is a good indicator of any atherosclerotic plaque buildup. For a patient with AF, a CT angiogram is preferred as it accurately shows the interior of the heart [21]. Through this test, common AF manifestations like fast/disorganized atrial activation may be observed. An echo operates by implementing sound waves to create real-time images of the patient's heart and can be useful in observing valve function and cardiac muscle health. In patients with AF, an echo will show how the heart contracts, and through that, observers will be able to notice how atrial contractions appear irregular and rapid [22]. An echo is accurate in displaying valve function and can show any abnormalities that may be associated with them, as well as with cardiac contractions.

Cardiac MRI has emerged as a valuable tool for interrogating the underlying substrate in AF patients. MRI uses a magnetic field to capture incoming radio waves from hydrogen atoms in various cells that respond to the magnification [23]. Like a CT scan, an MRI can provide highly accurate anatomical visualization. A cardiac MRI can additionally help analyze manifestations like atrial fibrosis and fat buildup around the heart walls. In addition to traditional MRI, four-dimensional flow (4D-flow) MRI is a very accurate and versatile way of visualizing and determining the size of biomarkers, including 3D stasis, vortices, changes in pressure, as well as flow distribution. 4D-flow MRI imaging helps achieve the precise visualization of the heart chambers, where manifestations of AF, including thrombus formations and hemodynamic efficiency, can be seen. The next section will introduce more in detail how new 4D-flow MRI approaches can accurately outline the progression of the AF.

2. Cardiovascular magnetic resonance for atrial fibrillation

In recent years, the innovation in interventional therapies and cardiac imaging for AF has motivated great interest and attention to a deeper understanding of the

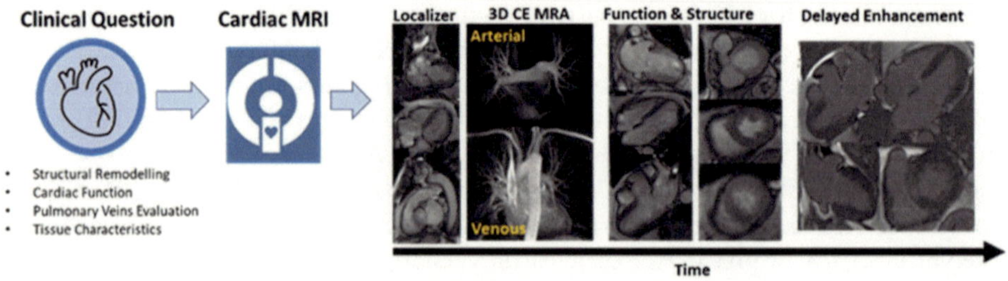

Figure 1.
Standard cardiac magnetic resonance imaging scan. Localizers facilitate the acquisition planning using anatomic images from the three directions of the heart. Heart landmarks are used to generate standard analysis planes views. Contrast-enhanced (CE) magnetic resonance angiogram (MRA) facilitates the assessment of the 3D LA structure and pulmonary veins anatomy. Standard cardiac cine imaging can be used for the assessment of the heart function and structure. Delayed enhancement images facilitate the tissue characterization of the heart. MRI: magnetic resonance imaging.

atrial anatomic structure and function. In addition, the innovations in 3D blood flow assessment have revealed a new light in the effect that AF has on heart hemodynamics. The standard cardiac magnetic resonance protocol for AF aims to provide a detailed assessment of LV/LA structure and function (**Figure 1**) [24].

There is a clinical indication for pulmonary vein assessment preablation procedure [24–26]. The postablation imaging remains optional. The LA has a highly complex structure with close interaction between the anatomical, structural, and functional aspects. The LA imaging assessment aims to characterize the two parts of the LA: the posterior-superior inflow (venous) and the anteroinferior outflow (vestibular). Both the contrast-enhanced (CE) and noncontrast techniques can be used for the evaluation of the pulmonary veins. Noncontrast cardiac-triggered imaging with respiratory navigation-gating balanced steady-state free precession (bSSFP) can provide high-quality images in a short time for assessing the basic clinical questions [27]. CE can be performed with both the extracellular and blood pool contrast agents. The intravascular half-time life of the extracellular chelates ranges between 60 and 120 s [28]. The extracellular contrast agents have a rapid leakage into the interstitial space that reduces the enhancement of both arteries and veins shortly after injection. To obtain reasonable-quality images, it is recommended to initiate the acquisition immediately after the first pass of the contrast agent. A more recent strategy includes the use of ferumoxytol as blood pool agent, which has a much longer half-time life, facilitating ultrahigh spatial resolution of both the arterial and the venous systems [29]. The voxel size difference achieved with ferumoxytol is one order of magnitude smaller compared with traditional acquisitions [30]. It is recommended to perform the breath-held 3D CE angiogram in the coronal projection encompassing the pulmonary veins and LA [24]. The use of an oblique plane centering the pulmonary veins can reduce the slab thickness but will lead to less coverage of the LA. When the patient has irregular rhythm, the ECG gating should be synchronized with systole. Three volumetric acquisitions are recommended: (1) precontrast, (2) first pass, and (3) after contrast administration. The precontrast acquisition serves as a reference for subtraction. A time-resolved multiphase (acquisition and contrast started simultaneously) angiogram can provide an isolated pulmonary phase image for reconstruction and integration with common ablation mapping software. Contrast should be injected at a 2–3-mL/s rate for an optimal result. Image slice thickness can be 1–2 mm with an in-plane resolution of 1–1.5 mm. An isotropic configuration is

DOI: http://dx.doi.org/10.5772/intechopen.105498

preferred (i.e., 1 × 1 × 1 mm). A slab of 60–80 slices typically covers a normal heart, and the number of slices can be increased to encompass the volume of interest. Standard 2D phase-contrast acquisitions can be added to quantify flow through each pulmonary vein. Late-gadolinium enhancement can also be added to assess the LA wall for fibrosis [31].

3. Advanced hemodynamic assessment in AF using 4D-flow

Four-dimensional flow (4D-flow) has been developed to achieve a comprehensive acquisition of blood flow through the heart [32, 33]. Phase-contrast flow-encoding acquisitions are performed in all three spatial dimensions of space and time along the cardiac cycle (3D + time = 4D). This technique has existed since earlier 1990s; however, computational and hardware limitations limited its clinical applicability [34]. During the last decade, both computational power and hardware development have allowed for a realistic integration into clinical settings. In recent years, a scientific consensus and acquisition recommendations have been published with the purpose of standardizing the acquisition and analysis of 4D-flow data [35–37]. Acquisition parameters are optimized to provide the best possible imaging accuracy in each protocol. For AF imaging, the slab acquisition can be sagittal or axial with whole-heart coverage using isotropic spatial resolution (2–2.5 mm). Retrospectively ECG-gated acquisition with 30 phases is advised for adequate coverage of the cardiac cycle. A respiratory navigator can be used to reduce respiratory motion. Acceleration methods, such as parallel imaging or compressed sensing, can be used to achieve an acquisition time between 5 and 10 min. A sample of acquisition is illustrated in **Figure 2**.

There have been efforts to quantify 4D-flow measurements to improve diagnosis and evaluation of disease and risk assessment of AF (**Table 1**).

An initial application of 4D-flow is the generation of phase-contrast angiogram (PC MRA), which can be obtained by multiplying the velocity magnitude and the cine magnitude volumes. One of the advantages of PC MRA versus the CE MRA is that it can be obtained without contrast and allow us to obtain comparable anatomic characterization for the pulmonary veins (**Figure 3**). One limitation is the limited characterization of the LAA. The primary method of characterizing hemodynamics in LA, from 3D blood flow velocities, is to take an average from all voxels through a whole

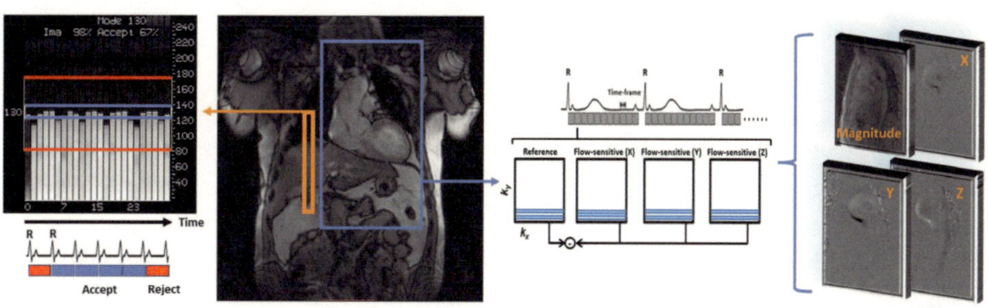

Figure 2.
Acquisition planning of 4D-flow. Region of interest covers the whole heart, as illustrated by the blue rectangle. The acquisition requires electrocardiogram gating and respiratory control, as it is shown by the small orange rectangle. Velocity encoding in each direction of the volume of interest is used to obtain velocity phases, which are subtracted from encoding reference to calculate blood flow velocities within the volume (X, Y, Z). The cardiac cycle average magnitude facilitates the anatomic visualization of the heart.

Study	Cohorts size (n)	Flow parameters	Findings
Fluckiger et al. (2013) [38]	Paroxysmal AF (n = 6), Persistent AF (n = 4), Controls (n = 19)	Mean velocity	Mean velocity decrease in persistent AF.
Markl et al. (2016) [39]	AF sinus rhythm (n = 42), AF in fibrillation (n = 39), Young controls (n = 10), Adult controls (n = 20)	LA peak velocity, LA time-to-peak velocity, LA flow stasis	LA peak velocity increases during fibrillation. LA flow stasis increases during sinus rhythm and fibrillation.
Lee et al. (2016) [40]	AF (n = 40), Young controls (n = 24), Adult controls (n = 20)	LA mean velocity, LA median velocity, and LA peak velocity	LA mean and median velocities significantly decrease. CHA_2DS_2-VASc score inversely correlated with mean, median, and peak velocity.
Markl et al. (2016) [41]	AF-sinus (n = 30), AF-afib (n = 30), Controls (n = 15)	Mean and peak velocity, LA and LAA Stasis	Individual variability of flow patterns in AF patients, despite the same CHA_2DS_2-VASc score. CHA_2DS_2-VASc is positively associated with LA flow stasis, but negatively with LA velocity.
Garcia et al. (2020) [42]	Paroxysmal AF (n = 45), Adult controls (n = 15)	Mean, median, and peak LA velocities, pulmonary vein peak velocity, LA blood flow stasis, and vortex size	Mean and median LA velocity decreases. Pulmonary veins peak velocity decreases. LA blood flow stasis increases. LA vortex size increases and correlates with CHA_2DS_2-VASc score.
Kim et al. (2020) [43]	Paroxysmal AF (n = 28), Controls (n = 10)	LA peak velocity, LV delayed ejection, LV residual volume, valve regurgitation	LV residual volume decreases. LV delayed ejection increases.
Demirkiran et al. (2021) [44]	Paroxysmal AF (n = 10), Adult controls (n = 5)	LA velocity (mean and peak), LA and LAA blood flow stasis, LA KE (mean and peak)	LA mean/peak velocities decreases. LA and LAA blood flow stasis increases. Mean and peak KE decreases.
Spartera et al. (2021) [45]	AF-afib (n = 22), AF-sinus (n = 64)	Mean and peak velocity, blood flow stasis, LA vorticity, LA vortex volume	LA peak velocity and vorticity showed reproducibility, stability, and demonstrated similar interval-scan variability
Spartera et al. (2021) [46]	Persistent AF (n = 37), High risk controls (n = 35), Low risk controls (n = 23)	Velocity (mean and peak), vortex to LA volume ratio, vorticity	Regardless of a history of AF, the high-risk group display altered flow characteristics

LA: left atrium; LAA: left atrial appendage; AF: atrial fibrillation; AF-sinus: previous history of AF, but in sinus rhythm at time of imaging; AF-afib: in AF at the time of imaging; KE: kinetic energy; CHA_2DS_2-VASc: stroke risk stratification system that accounts for the patient history of congestive heart failure, hypertension, age > 75 years, diabetes mellitus, stroke, vascular disease, age between 64 and 75 years, and sex.

Table 1.
Summary of 4D-flow studies on AF. Flow parameter comparisons between healthy controls and AF patients have revealed consistent differences, such as reduced flow velocity and increased stasis. In recent years, the interest in novel flow parameters and association with risk factors are grown.

cardiac cycle or peak velocity. Although there is some contradiction between studies, most of the recent studies characterizing AF blood flow with relatively large cohorts agree that there is a significant decrease in mean and peak flow velocity in LA, even in paroxysmal AF patients with sinus rhythm [39–42, 44]. Most notably, the increase

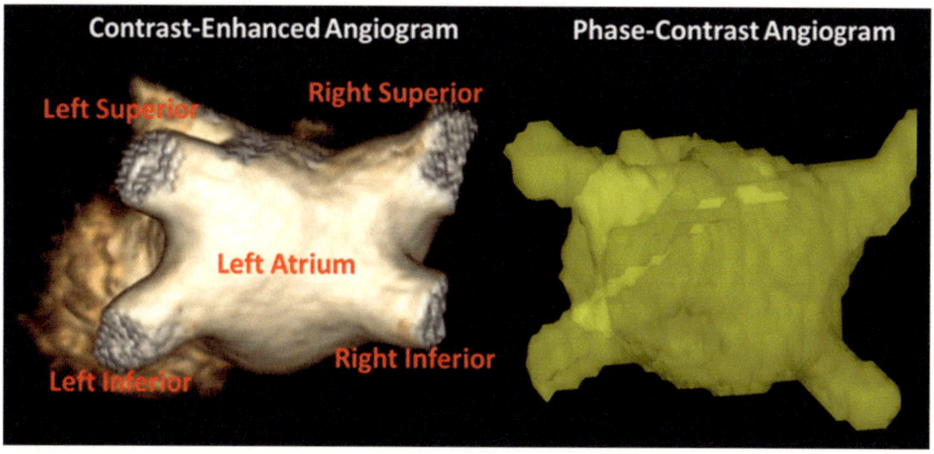

Figure 3.
Comparison of contrast-enhanced angiogram and phase-contrast angiogram in a patient with atrial fibrillation. Contrast-enhanced (CE) acquisition requires the use of an agent to depict the left atrial anatomy. Phase-contrast (PC) angiograms derived from 4D-flow do not require the use of a contrast agent. CE angiogram benefits from a higher spatial resolution (1 mm isotropic) than PC angiogram (~2.5 mm isotropic). Both the acquisitions are useful to characterize the pulmonary vein structure.

in CHA_2DS_2-VASc score has been associated with reduced mean LA velocity [40, 41], which suggests that 4D-flow measurement may be able to improve risk assessment.

Kinetic energy, which is proportional to the mean square of velocity, was also markedly lower in AF patients than in controls [44]. Similarly, energy loss is also reduced (**Figure 4**). Left atrial flow stasis map proposed by Markl et al. [39] focuses on the flow

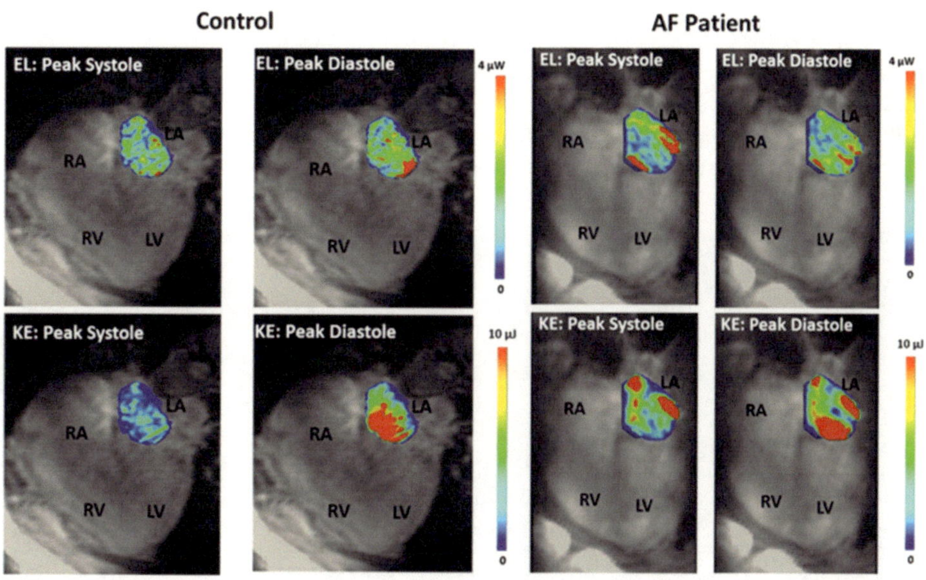

Figure 4.
Kinetic energy and energy loss. On the left, a control quantification sample of energy loss (EL) and kinetic energy (KE) in the left atrium (LA). On the right, a preablation atrial fibrillation (AF) patient. Local energy differences are mostly generated from the pulmonary veins during inflow, as it is showed by the red regions. RA: right atrium; RV: right ventricle; LV: left ventricle.

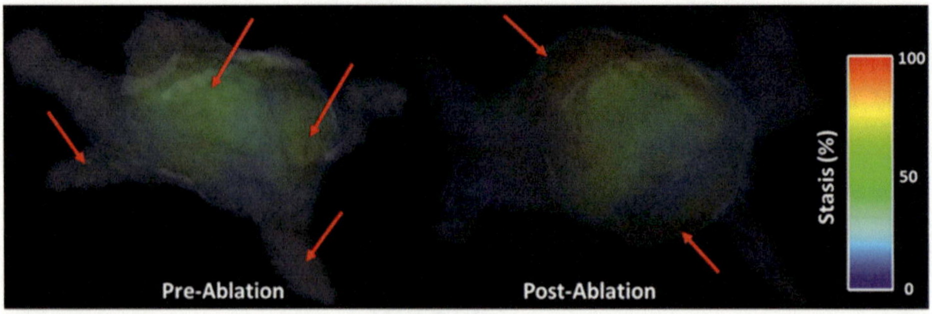

Figure 5.
Left atrial stasis maps. Sample of a patient 3D stasis map pre- and postablation showing regions with elevated stasis (red arrows). Larger stasis regions are indicators of possible thrombus formation. The region near the left atrial appendage typically shows elevated stasis after ablation.

stagnation at individual voxel. This method counts the number of time frames under threshold velocity (0.1 m/s) at each voxel, which is supposed to increase the chance of thrombosis. The result can be shown as a map projected on the MRA image as well as the average ratio relative to the one whole heart cycle. Several studies have consistently reported flow stasis to be elevated in AF patients both in sinus rhythm and in fibrillation [39, 41, 42, 45]. An example of flow stasis is displayed in **Figure 5**.

In addition, flow patterns through the pulmonary vein into the LA have been studied [42]. The 3D asymmetrical configuration of the systemic pulmonary veins allows the development of vortical flow patterns during early diastolic LV filling while avoiding/reducing blood stasis [42]. AF patients often show LA inflow fragmentation and vortex formation in the LA (see **Figure 6**). Increment of vortex size can be observed in paroxysmal AF, and it is associated with higher risk score. Similarly, decreased LA velocity and increased LA blood flow stasis have also been reported in the LAA [41, 44]. However, 4D-flow MRI special resolution may not facilitate the accurate segmentation the LAA [35]. Despite the latter, 4D-flow parameters have shown excellent reliability and reproducibility in AF patients [45]. LA peak velocity and vorticity were found to be more reproducible and independent of physiological biomarkers than LA mean velocity, LA vortex volume, and blood flow stasis.

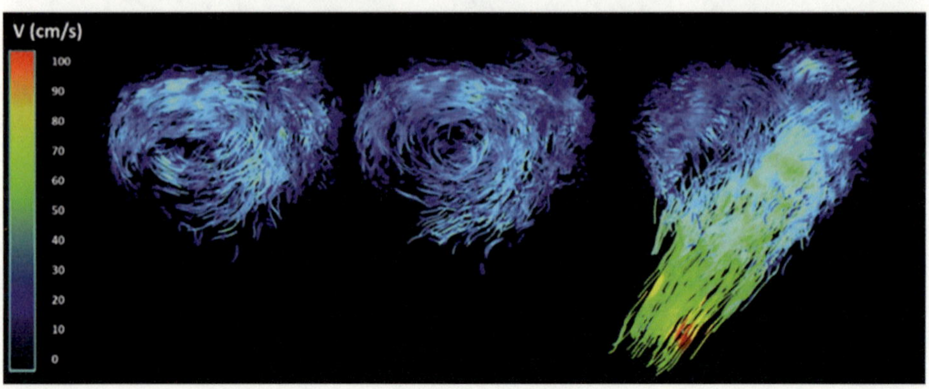

Figure 6.
Evolution of atrial vortex formation in atrial fibrillation. A vortex typically forms during left atrial inflow and tends to disappear during ejection. However, in atrial fibrillation patients, small vortices remain in the atrium during the cardiac cycle.

There was an approach to associate risk factors with LA flow characteristics [46]. This study presented patients with moderate to high CHA_2DS_2-VASc scores have impaired LA flow parameters even though they have restored from arrhythmia or have no AF history. Recently, a novel sequence to evaluate 3D hemodynamics with a fully self-gated and free-running sequence, called 5D flow, has been proposed [47]. This method extracts cardiac and respiratory signals from SI projection signals, eliminating the need for ECG gating, and adds the respiratory phase as the fifth dimension by sorting acquired scan lines according to respiratory signal. This method can be extended to be used in AF patients by replacing the respiratory dimension with the RR length dimension to tackle the variability of arrhythmic heartbeats [48]. The study successfully found a correlation between flow parameters and AF burden with reasonable scan time (<10 min).

4. Conclusion

In conclusion, advances in cardiac magnetic resonance imaging can facilitate the assessment of cardiac function and left atrial structure. This chapter aimed to introduce a standard cardiac MRI protocol for atrial fibrillation. Advanced hemodynamics using 4D-flow can improve the assessment of the left atrium flow patterns and efficiency throughout the cardiac cycle. Novel flow biomarkers such as 3D stasis, kinetic energy, or vortex formation may unmask the presence of LA/LV disease in atrial fibrillation.

Acknowledgements

The authors were supported by The University of Calgary, URGC SEM #1054341 and JG start-up funding. Research unrestricted funding was also provided by The Libin Cardiovascular Institute and Siemens Healthineers. JG acknowledges the Natural Science and Engineering Research Council of Canada, grants RGPIN-2020-04549 and DGECR-2020-00204.

Conflict of interest

The authors have no conflict of interest.

Author details

Mankarman Ghuman, Hansuk Kim, Hana Sheitt and Julio Garcia*
University of Calgary, Calgary, Alberta, Canada

*Address all correspondence to: julio.garciaflores@ucalgary.ca

References

[1] January CT, Wann LS, Alpert JS, et al. 2014 AHA/ACC/HRS guideline for the management of patients with atrial fibrillation: A report of the American college of cardiology/American heart association task force on practice guidelines and the heart rhythm society. Journal of the American College of Cardiology. 2014;**64**(21):e1-e76

[2] Andrade JG, Aguilar M, Atzema C, et al. The 2020 Canadian cardiovascular society/Canadian heart rhythm society comprehensive guidelines for the management of atrial fibrillation. The Canadian Journal of Cardiology. 2020;**36**(12):1847-1948

[3] Staerk L, Wang B, Preis SR, et al. Lifetime risk of atrial fibrillation according to optimal, borderline, or elevated levels of risk factors: Cohort study based on longitudinal data from the Framingham Heart Study. BMJ. 2018;**26**:k1453. Available from: https://www.bmj.com/lookup/doi/10.1136/bmj.k1453

[4] Michaud GF, Stevenson WG. Atrial fibrillation. The New England Journal of Medicine. 2021;**384**(4):353-361. Available from: http://www.nejm.org/doi/10.1056/NEJMcp2023658

[5] Spartalis M, Tzatzaki E, Spartalis E, et al. Pathophysiology and current evidence for detection of dyssynchrony. Cardiology Research. 2017;**8**(5):179-183. Available from: http://www.cardiologyres.org/index.php/Cardiologyres/article/view/598

[6] Chamberlain AM, Agarwal SK, Folsom AR, et al. Smoking and incidence of atrial fibrillation: Results from the Atherosclerosis Risk in Communities (ARIC) study. Heart Rhythm. 2011;**8**(8):1160-1166. Available from: https://linkinghub.elsevier.com/retrieve/pii/S1547527111003055

[7] Wang EY, Hulme OL, Khurshid S, et al. Initial precipitants and recurrence of atrial fibrillation. Circulation. Arrhythmia and Electrophysiology. 2020;**13**:e007716. Available from: https://www.ahajournals.org/doi/10.1161/CIRCEP.119.007716

[8] Turhan S, Ulas Ozcan O, Erol C. Imaging of intracardiac thrombus. Cor et Vasa. 2013;**55**(2):e176-e183. Available from: http://e-coretvasa.cz/doi/10.1016/j.crvasa.2013.02.005.html

[9] Furie B, Furie BC. Mechanisms of thrombus formation. The New England Journal of Medicine. 2008;**359**(9):938-949. Available from: http://www.nejm.org/doi/abs/10.1056/NEJMra0801082

[10] Clark DM, Plumb VJ, Epstein AE, Kay GN. Hemodynamic effects of an irregular sequence of ventricular cycle lengths during atrial fibrillation. Journal of the American College of Cardiology. 1997;**30**(4):1039-1045. Available from: https://linkinghub.elsevier.com/retrieve/pii/S0735109797002544

[11] Kamel H, Okin PM, Elkind MSV, Iadecola C. Atrial fibrillation and mechanisms of stroke. Stroke. 2016;**47**(3):895-900. Available from: https://www.ahajournals.org/doi/10.1161/STROKEAHA.115.012004

[12] Lee E, Choi E-K, Han K-D, et al. Mortality and causes of death in patients with atrial fibrillation: A nationwide population-based study. PLoS One. 2018;**13**(12):e0209687. DOI: 10.1371/journal.pone.0209687

[13] Benjamin EJ, Wolf PA, D'Agostino RB, Silbershatz H, Kannel WB, Levy D. Impact of atrial fibrillation on the risk

of death: The framingham heart study. Circulation. 1998;**98**(10):946-952. Available from: http://www.ncbi.nlm.nih.gov/pubmed/9737513

[14] Yamamoto M, Seo Y, Kawamatsu N, et al. Complex left atrial appendage morphology and left atrial appendage thrombus formation in patients with atrial fibrillation. Circulation. Cardiovascular Imaging. 2014;**7**(2): 337-343. Available from: https://www.ahajournals.org/doi/10.1161/CIRCIMAGING.113.001317

[15] Pamukcu B, Lip GYH, Lane DA. Simplifying stroke risk stratification in atrial fibrillation patients: Implications of the CHA2DS2-VASc risk stratification scores. Age and Ageing. 2010;**39**(5):533-535

[16] Dulli DA, Stanko H, Levine RL. Atrial fibrillation is associated with severe acute ischemic stroke. Neuroepidemiology. 2003;**22**(2):118-123. Available from: https://www.karger.com/Article/FullText/68743

[17] Habibi M, Lima JAC, Khurram IM, et al. Association of left atrial function and left atrial enhancement in patients with atrial fibrillation. Circulation: Cardiovascular Imaging. 2015;**8**:e002769. Available from: https://www.ahajournals.org/doi/10.1161/CIRCIMAGING.114.002769

[18] Blum S, Aeschbacher S, Meyre P, et al. Incidence and predictors of atrial fibrillation progression. Journal of the American Heart Association. 2019;**8**:e012554. Available from: https://www.ahajournals.org/doi/10.1161/JAHA.119.012554

[19] Couceiro R, Carvalho P, Henriques J, Antunes M, Harris M, Habetha J. Detection of atrial fibrillation using model-based ECG analysis. In: 2008 19th International Conference on Pattern Recognition. IEEE; 2008. p. 1-5. Available from: http://ieeexplore.ieee.org/document/4761755/

[20] Harris K, Edwards D, Mant J. How can we best detect atrial fibrillation? The Journal of the Royal College of Physicians of Edinburgh. 2012;**42**(Suppl 1):5-22. Available from: http://www.ncbi.nlm.nih.gov/pubmed/22518390

[21] Vorre MM, Abdulla J. Diagnostic accuracy and radiation dose of CT coronary angiography in atrial fibrillation: Systematic review and meta-analysis. Radiology. 2013;**267**(2):376-386. Available from: http://pubs.rsna.org/doi/10.1148/radiol.13121224

[22] Troughton RW. The role of echocardiography in atrial fibrillation and cardioversion. Heart. 2003;**89**(12):1447-1454. Available from: https://heart.bmj.com/lookup/doi/10.1136/heart.89.12.1447

[23] Pfeiffer MP, Biederman RWW. Cardiac MRI: A general overview with emphasis on current use and indications. The Medical Clinics of North America. 2015;**99**(4):849-861. Available from: https://linkinghub.elsevier.com/retrieve/pii/S0025712515000449

[24] Kramer CM, Barkhausen J, Bucciarelli-Ducci C, Flamm SD, Kim RJ, Nagel E. Standardized cardiovascular magnetic resonance imaging (CMR) protocols: 2020 update. Journal of Cardiovascular Magnetic Resonance. 2020;**22**(1):17. Available from: https://jcmr-online.biomedcentral.com/articles/10.1186/s12968-020-00607-1

[25] Leiner T, Bogaert J, Friedrich MG, et al. SCMR Position Paper (2020) on clinical indications for cardiovascular magnetic resonance. Journal of Cardiovascular Magnetic Resonance. 2020;**22**(1):76. Available from:

https://jcmr-online.biomedcentral.com/articles/10.1186/s12968-020-00682-4

[26] AlJaroudi WA, Saliba WS, Wazni OM, Jaber WA. Role of cardiac computed tomography and cardiovascular magnetic resonance imaging in guiding management and treatment of patients with atrial fibrillation: State of the art review. Journal of Nuclear Cardiology. 2013;**20**(3):426-442. Available from: http://link.springer.com/10.1007/s12350-013-9689-z

[27] Kim CY, Bashir MR, Heye T, Dale BM, Nichols HL, Merkle EM. Respiratory-gated noncontrast SPACE MR angiography sequence at 3T for evaluation of the central veins of the chest: A feasibility study. Journal of Magnetic Resonance Imaging. 2015;**41**(1):67-73. Available from: https://onlinelibrary.wiley.com/doi/10.1002/jmri.24540

[28] Aime S, Caravan P. Biodistribution of gadolinium-based contrast agents, including gadolinium deposition. Journal of Magnetic Resonance Imaging. 2009;**30**(6):1259-1267. Available from: https://onlinelibrary.wiley.com/doi/10.1002/jmri.21969

[29] Finn JP, Nguyen K-L, Han F, et al. Cardiovascular MRI with ferumoxytol. Clinical Radiology. 2016;**71**(8):796-806. Available from: https://linkinghub.elsevier.com/retrieve/pii/S0009926016300083

[30] Nguyen K-L, Han F, Zhou Z, et al. 4D MUSIC CMR: Value-based imaging of neonates and infants with congenital heart disease. Journal of Cardiovascular Magnetic Resonance. 2017;**19**(1):40. Available from: https://jcmr-online.biomedcentral.com/articles/10.1186/s12968-017-0352-8

[31] De Sensi F, Penela D, Soto-Iglesias D, Berruezo A, Limbruno U. Imaging techniques for the study of fibrosis in atrial fibrillation ablation: From molecular mechanisms to therapeutical perspectives. Journal of Clinical Medicine. 2021;**10**(11):2277. Available from: https://www.mdpi.com/2077-0383/10/11/2277

[32] Markl M, Chan FP, Alley MT, et al. Time-resolved three-dimensional phase-contrast MRI. Journal of Magnetic Resonance Imaging. 2003;**17**(4):499-506. Available from: http://www.ncbi.nlm.nih.gov/pubmed/12655592

[33] Wigström L, Sjöqvist L, Wranne B. Temporally resolved 3D phase-contrast imaging. Magnetic Resonance in Medicine. 1996;**36**(5):800-803. Available from: http://www.ncbi.nlm.nih.gov/pubmed/8916033

[34] Kilner PJ, Manzara CC, Mohiaddin RH, et al. Magnetic resonance jet velocity mapping in mitral and aortic valve stenosis. Circulation. 1993;**87**(4):1239-1248 Available from: http://www.ncbi.nlm.nih.gov/pubmed/8462150

[35] Dyverfeldt P, Bissell M, Barker AJ, et al. 4D flow cardiovascular magnetic resonance consensus statement. Journal of Cardiovascular Magnetic Resonance. 2015;**17**(1):72

[36] Garcia J, Barker AJ, Markl M. The role of imaging of flow patterns by 4D Flow MRI in aortic stenosis. JACC: Cardiovascular Imaging. 2019;**12**(2):252-266. Available from: https://linkinghub.elsevier.com/retrieve/pii/S1936878X1831115X

[37] Zhong L, Schrauben EM, Garcia J, et al. Intracardiac 4D flow MRI in congenital heart disease: Recommendations on behalf of the

ISMRM flow & motion study group. Journal of Magnetic Resonance Imaging. 2019;**50**(3):677-681

[38] Fluckiger JU, Goldberger JJ, Lee DC, et al. Left atrial flow velocity distribution and flow coherence using four-dimensional FLOW MRI: A pilot study investigating the impact of age and Pre- and Postintervention atrial fibrillation on atrial hemodynamics. Journal of Magnetic Resonance Imaging. 2013;**38**(3):580-587

[39] Markl M, Lee DC, Ng J, Carr M, Carr J, Goldberger JJ. Left Atrial 4-dimensional flow magnetic resonance imaging: Stasis and velocity mapping in patients with atrial fibrillation. Investigative Radiology. 2016;**51**(3):147-154

[40] Lee DC, Markl M, Ng J, et al. Three-dimensional left atrial blood flow characteristics in patients with atrial fibrillation assessed by 4D flow CMR. European Heart Journal Cardiovascular Imaging. 2016;**17**(11):1259-1268

[41] Markl M, Lee DC, Furiasse N, et al. Left atrial and left atrial appendage 4D blood flow dynamics in atrial fibrillation. Circulation. Cardiovascular Imaging. 2016;**9**(9):e004984

[42] Garcia J, Sheitt H, Bristow MS, et al. Left atrial vortex size and velocity distributions by 4D flow MRI in patients with paroxysmal atrial fibrillation: Associations with age and CHA2 DS2 -VASc risk score. Journal of Magnetic Resonance Imaging. 2020;**51**(3):871-884

[43] Kim H, Sheitt H, Jamalidinan F, Wilton S, White J, Garcia J. Left ventricular flow analysis in atrial fibrillation. 42nd Annual International Conference of the IEEE Engineering in Medicine & Biology Society (EMBC). IEEE. 2020;**2020**:1182-1185

[44] Demirkiran A, Amier RP, Hofman MBM, et al. Altered left atrial 4D flow characteristics in patients with paroxysmal atrial fibrillation in the absence of apparent remodeling. Scientific Reports. 2021;**11**(1):5965

[45] Spartera M, Pessoa-Amorim G, Stracquadanio A, et al. Left atrial 4D flow cardiovascular magnetic resonance: A reproducibility study in sinus rhythm and atrial fibrillation. Journal of Cardiovascular Magnetic Resonance. 2021;**23**(1):29

[46] Spartera M, Stracquadanio A, Pessoa-Amorim G, et al. The impact of atrial fibrillation and stroke risk factors on left atrial blood flow characteristics. European Heart Journal Cardiovascular Imaging. 2021;**23**(1):115-123

[47] Ma LE, Yerly J, Piccini D, et al. 5d flow mri: A fully self-gated, free-running framework for cardiac and respiratory motion–resolved 3d hemodynamics. Radiology: Cardiothoracic Imaging. 12 Nov 2020;**2**(6):e200219. DOI: 10.1148/ryct.2020200219

[48] Ma L, Yerly J, Di Sopra L, et al. Using 5D flow MRI to decode the effects of rhythm on left atrial 3D flow dynamics in patients with atrial fibrillation. Magnetic Resonance in Medicine. 2021;**85**(6):3125-3139. Available from: http://www.ncbi.nlm.nih.gov/pubmed/33400296

Chapter 5

Dual Antiplatelet Therapy

Edidiong Orok, Funmilayo Adeniyi and Oluwole Akawa

Abstract

Antiplatelet agents have been utilized to enhance outcomes in patients with acute coronary syndrome for decades and are increasingly valued for their antithrombotic as well as anti-inflammatory characteristics. Dual antiplatelet therapy (DAPT) is a combination of aspirin and a P2Y12 inhibitor. Different modes of action are employed by these drugs. Aspirin is an anti-inflammatory medication that also has antioxidant characteristics, while P2Y12 inhibitors act by inhibiting thrombocytes activation/ aggregation. There are two types of P2Y12 inhibitors: thienopyridines and nucleoside/ nucleotide compounds. Nucleoside/nucleotide derivatives are reversible direct-acting P2Y12 receptor antagonists that do not need hepatic metabolism, whereas thienopyridines are competitive and irreversible P2Y12 inhibitors. In patients with acute coronary syndrome or undergoing percutaneous coronary intervention for stable coronary artery disease, dual antiplatelet therapy, which contains aspirin and a P2Y12 receptor inhibitor, has consistently been shown to reduce recurrent major adverse cardiovascular events compared to aspirin monotherapy, but at the cost of an increased risk of major bleeding. This chapter is meant to elaborate on dual antiplatelet therapy highlighting the current guidelines and recent evidences on the indications, dosing, and duration of treatment using dual antiplatelet therapy.

Keywords: dual antiplatelet therapy, aspirin, P2Y12 inhibitors, acute coronary syndrome, coronary artery disease

1. Introduction

Because of a global change in illness and death from infectious to noninfectious causes during the 20th century, life expectancy doubled and global population quadrupled [1]. Cardiovascular diseases (CVDs) have surpassed cancer as the main cause of mortality, with low- and middle-income countries bearing the brunt of the burden [2].

In 2015, the United States spent more than $200 billion on heart problems, including related medications and health-care services [3]. In 2017, the American Cardiology Association reported that more than 360,000 persons were diagnosed with coronary heart disease [4].

The principal therapy for preventing arterial thrombosis in CVD patients is platelet inhibitors [5, 6]. Dual antiplatelet therapy (DAPT) with aspirin and a P2Y12 inhibitor is the standard medical treatment for patients with acute coronary syndrome (ACS) and those undergoing percutaneous coronary intervention (PCI) with an intracoronary stent [6].

Every year, about 1.2 million patients get DAPT after receiving a drug-eluting stent (DES). DAPT is used for a variety of cardiologic, neurologic, and surgical indications where the need to prevent thromboembolic events outweighs the risk of bleeding [7, 8]. DAPT is widely used to treat thrombotic stroke, coronary artery disease (CAD), peripheral vascular diseases, and transient ischemic attack (TIA). When compared to aspirin alone, DAPT with aspirin and clopidogrel has been shown to enhance clinical outcomes in patients with acute coronary syndrome or PCI [9, 10].

Despite the effectiveness of DAPT in preventing primary and subsequent myocardial infarction (MI) and stroke, there is an increased associated risk of spontaneous intracerebral hemorrhage (ICH) [11]. Interestingly, in-hospital mortality is greater in patients with ICH who are on DAPT compared to other antiplatelet agents [12, 13]. The goal of achieving efficient antiplatelet activity while avoiding gastrointestinal (GI) injury and bleeding has become a key focus in the management of thrombotic disease patients. This chapter is meant to explore on dual antiplatelet therapy highlighting the current guidelines and recent evidences on the indications, dosing, and duration of treatment using dual antiplatelet therapy.

2. Mechanisms of action of the components of DAPT

DAPT comprises of aspirin together with a P2Y12 inhibitor. These agents have different mechanisms of actions. This section will focus solely on the mechanism of action related to antithrombotic effects of dual antiplatelet therapy.

2.1 Mechanism of action of aspirin

Aspirin is an anti-inflammatory drug, which possesses both anti-inflammatory and antioxidant properties [14]. The primary mechanism of action of aspirin is centered on the irreversible inhibition of cyclooxygenase (COX 1) enzyme, thus preventing the conversion of arachidonic acid into prostaglandin G2 and prostaglandin H2, subsequently inhibiting thromboxane A2 synthesis. Aspirin acetylates and forms a covalent bond with serine residues in COX active site at position 529, thus inhibiting cox 1 enzyme [15, 16]. Other activities of aspirin include mitochondrial oxidative phosphorylation and modulation of NF-KB signals [14].

2.2 Mechanism of action of P2Y12 inhibitors

P2Y12 inhibitors, otherwise known as P2Y12 antagonists, act by blocking P2Y12 adenosine diphosphate (ADP) receptors on platelet surface membrane, subsequently inhibiting thrombocyte activation/aggregation [17]. P2Y12 inhibitors can be classified into two groups: thienopyridines and nucleoside/nucleotide derivatives [16].

Thienopyridines are competitive and irreversible P2Y12 inhibitors [16]. Drugs in this class can be further subdivided into three generations: first-, second-, and third-generation thienopyridines.

Ticlopidine is a first-generation thienopyridines that was withdrawn due to major side effects such as GI disorders, cytopenia, and allergies. Clopidogrel is a prodrug of second-generation thienopyridine derivatives, which is a drug of first choice in DAPT. Clopidogrel active metabolite binds to P2Y12 receptor to form an irreversible covalent bond, which inhibits ADP-dependent platelet activation and aggregation [18]. Dual antiplatelet therapy with aspirin and clopidogrel has been associated with more than 3% platelet reactivity [19] and 10% ischemic occurrences after 12 months of treatment.

Third-generation thienopyridine (prasugrel) was developed with rapid absorption and higher bioavailability than clopidogrel [16, 18].

Some drugs in this class are mainly reversible P2Y12 inhibitors such as ticagrelor and cangrelor. Ticagrelor is a more potent, efficacious, and fast acting P2Y12 inhibitor when compared with other P2Y12 inhibitors such as clopidogrel and prasugrel [20]. Ticagrelor acts by binding to P2Y12 receptor site other than the ADP binding site. In addition, ticagrelor binds to equilibrative nucleoside transporter 1 (ENT 1) in platelets and red blood cells to block the reuptake of adenosine [21].

The P2Y12 inhibitors have peculiar features, advantages and disadvantages, as well as adverse effects. These effects have been summarized in **Table 1**.

P2Y12 inhibitor	Advantages	Disadvantages	Adverse effects
Clopidogrel	• First drug of choice among P2Y12 inhibitors • DAPT with clopidogrel is efficient in preventing MACE • Prevents the risk of thrombotic complications in patients with AF that are undergoing PCI • Highly effective in secondary prevention of cardiovascular and cerebrovascular events • Greatest efficacy in patients undergoing thrombolysis • Once-daily dosing • Quite affordable	• Slow onset of antiplatelet effect. • High susceptibility to genetic variation and drug–drug interactions • Variability of response with a poor response associated with increased risk of thrombosis. • High platelet reactivity especially in diabetic patients subsequently leading to impaired antiplatelet response. • High risk of MACE in patients with vascular risk factors receiving clopidogrel therapy.	• Jaundice • Seizures • Gastric ulceration • Bloody vomit • Haematuria • Slow or difficult speech • Muscle weakness • Dyspnea • Tachycardia • Pale skin
Ticagrelor	• More potent, efficacious and fast acting P2Y12 inhibitor when compared with other P2Y12 inhibitors • Reduction in ischemic event rates unlike clopidogrel • Rapid and extensive platelet inhibition • Fast onset of effect and Reversible inhibition • Less susceptible to genetic variation and drug–drug interactions • Prevents non-fatal MI, ischaemic CVS events, stroke and other CVS related death	• Low bioavailability. • Increased risk of non–CABG surgery bleeding when compared with clopidogrel • Twice-daily dosing • It is expensive	• Dyspnea at rest, after exercise • Chest pain • Bleeding risk • Tachycardia, bradycardia or irregular heartbeat • Edema of the face, throat, tongue, lips, and eyes • Rashes

P2Y12 inhibitor	Advantages	Disadvantages	Adverse effects
Prasugrel	• Rapid absorption and higher bioavailability than clopidogrel • Lesser ischemic event rates following PCI unlike clopidogrel • Better efficacy in patients with diabetes and STEMI • Once-daily dosing • Fast and extensive platelet inhibition	• High risk of major bleeding, especially in patients undergoing CABG surgery • It is expensive	• Dyspnea • High bleeding risk • Purple patches on the skin • Muscle weakness • Cardiac arrhythmias • Headache • Jaundice • Confusion • Seizures • Stomach pain

KEY: *DAPT: dual antiplatelet therapy, MACE: major adverse cardiovascular events, ACS: acute coronary syndrome, PCI: percutaneous cardiovascular intervention, AF: atrial fibrillation, MI: myocardial infarction, CVS: cardiovascular, CABG: coronary artery bypass graft, STEMI-ST: elevation myocardial infarction.*
Source: *[22, 23].*

Table 1.
Advantages, disadvantages, and side effects of P2Y12 inhibitors.

3. Indications for DAPT

3.1 Atrial fibrillation

About 40% of patients with atrial fibrillation have a high risk of having CAD. DAPT prevents the risk of thrombotic complications in patients with atrial fibrillation that are undergoing percutaneous coronary intervention [24]. DAPT is preferable to triple therapy with an oral anticoagulant (OAC) due to low risk of bleeding and other thrombotic complications [24–26]. Clopidogrel is a drug of first choice; however, prasugrel and ticagrelor have been recently approved for treating patients with high ischemic risk and high risk of hemorrhage and stent thrombosis associated with clopidogrel [27].

However, prasugrel is contraindicated in patients undergoing treatment with aspirin and OAC due to the risk of hemorrhage [28].

3.2 Acute coronary syndrome

DAPT can be prescribed for prevention of ACS and other adverse cardiovascular (CVS) events. A combination of aspirin and ticagrelor or prasugrel is commonly recommended for treating patients with ACS within 6–12 months [29, 30]. DAPT is recommended for treating patients with ACS and atrial fibrillation who are at a risk of developing coronary artery disease, which may necessitate PCI with stents [31]. Clopidogrel can be replaced with ticagrelor in rare cases [32, 33]. Cangrelor, a potent intravenous P2Y12 inhibitor with fast onset of action, can be indicated for treating unconscious ACS patients on emergency who are unable to absorb an oral P2Y12 inhibitor [34].

3.3 Coronary artery disease

DAPT with aspirin and clopidogrel is recommended for patients with CAD in order to avert atherothrombotic events. In patients undergoing elective stent implantation, DAPT with aspirin and clopidogrel is usually recommended for 3–6 months [30, 35].

3.4 Myocardial infarction, ischemic events, and stroke

In previous years, DAPT with aspirin and clopidogrel or ticagrelor was formerly recommended for preventing recurrent stroke especially in patients with high risk of transient ischemic attack and noncardioembolic mild stroke [36]. However, DAPT has been found in previous studies to reduce the incidence of stroke and CVS-related death, thus making it effective for stroke prevention. Because DAPT reduces the risk of minor stroke and high transient ischemic attack in these patients, DAPT can be recommended in combination with aspirin and a P2Y12 inhibitor for acute treatment of patients with acute noncardioembolic minor ischemic stroke [37].

Novel and trending studies have compared the efficacy of other potent P2Y12 antagonist such as ticagrelor and prasugrel with clopidogrel especially in preventing nonfatal MI, ischemic CVS events, stroke, and other CVS-related death [38]. DAPT with aspirin and clopidogrel is also approved for treating patients with severe stenosis of the intracranial artery [39] and chronic symptomatic peripheral artery diseases (PADs) [40].

3.5 Transcatheter aortic valve implantation (TAVI), peripheral artery disease, atherosclerosis, and mechanical prosthesis

Dual antiplatelet therapy is indicated in patients on the line for transcatheter aortic valve implantation (TAVI) without high risk of hemorrhage for 3–6 months [17]. After revascularization, DAPT is usually indicated for 1–12 months in peripheral artery disease (PAD) patients [17]. It is worth to note that DAPT can be extended for more than 1 year in patients with atherosclerosis and mechanical prosthesis having high risk of coronary events [17].

3.6 Other indications of DAPT

DAPT can also be used in other nonconventional indications, which include diabetes, renal transplant, and carotid endarterectomy. In diabetes, DAPT consisting of aspirin and prasugrel or ticagrelor is indicated due to increased platelet reactivity [41]. DAPT administration reduces the risk of cardiovascular events in patients undergoing renal transplant. On the other hand, the risk of postoperative hemorrhage is increased with DAPT. Therefore, DAPT is strictly recommended for renal transplant patients with high risk of cardiovascular events [42]. DAPT can also be used for patients undergoing carotid endarterectomy [34].

4. Recent evidence and guidelines on DAPT use in patients

Antiplatelet therapy is an important pharmacological component in preventing atherothrombotic events. Aspirin, a widely used antiplatelet drug, has been found to reduce the risk of recurrent major adverse cardiovascular events (MACE) by around one-fifth [43]. However, the combination of antiplatelets has been reported to achieve better outcomes than the use of aspirin alone [10]. DAPT refers to a therapy that includes aspirin and a P2Y12 receptor inhibitor (clopidogrel, prasugrel, or ticagrelor). When compared to single antiplatelet medication, DAPT has been found to prevent recurrent major ischemic episodes in patients with ACS or undergoing PCI at the cost of an unavoidable increased risk of major bleeding [10]. Below are guidelines on the effective use of DAPT across various indications.

4.1 Use of DAPT after undergoing percutaneous coronary intervention

Clinical trials have shown that all the patients receiving PCI require DAPT as it reduces risk of short- and long-term thrombotic events when compared to aspirin. Current guidelines recommend a 6-month DAPT for patients with stable symptoms and a 12-month DAPT for those who have had an ACS [29].

Except for patients who have received a bioabsorbable drug-eluting stent, the clinical setting in which it occurs—stable or unstable—and the patient's bleeding risk are the two most important factors to consider when determining the DAPT duration following PCI. When feasible, extended (at least 12 months) and potent DAPT should be used for these individuals.

4.2 DAPT in stable coronary artery disease

Platelet inhibition is critical for the treatment and prevention of short- and long-term thrombotic events. The cyclooxygenase-1 inhibitor aspirin and the platelet adenosine diphosphate P2Y12 receptor inhibitors clopidogrel, prasugrel, and ticagrelor are all available as oral antiplatelet medicines for secondary prevention in patients with CAD. The more recent powerful P2Y12 platelet receptor inhibitors prasugrel and ticagrelor have been tested in individuals with ACS, whereas aspirin and clopidogrel have been studied across the entire range of CAD [44].

A 6-month DAPT time is advised for individuals with stable illness following PCI; however, this might be decreased based on the patient's bleeding risk or for safety considerations. The guidelines go beyond specifics and advocate for the use of metallic stents as a first-line therapy, even in patients who are only given a 1-month antiplatelet regimen for safety reasons [45, 46]. DAPT should be continued for 6 months in individuals who have had angioplasty with a drug-coated balloon. This guideline is based on the results of many clinical trials that employed empirical antiplatelet methods.

4.3 DAPT in acute coronary syndrome

The use of DAPT to inhibit platelet function after an acute coronary syndrome aims to reduce short- and long-term thrombotic consequences [47]. The stent protective effect of DAPT in the first weeks after percutaneous revascularization reduces the risk of stent thrombosis, a potentially fatal event caused by inflammation and endothelial damage associated with mechanical insult during PCI [48]. Long-term therapy has been demonstrated to reduce the risk of subsequent ischemia episodes caused not only by the culprit lesions/vessels, but also by the advancement of atherosclerosis, a phenomenon described as the "patient protective effect" [48].

Several antithrombotic medications have been proposed over time with the goal of offering the best thrombotic protection while minimizing hemorrhagic hazards. However, recent European guidelines advise the use of the two most modern and strong P2Y12 inhibitors (prasugrel and ticagrelor) in patients with or without PCI [49, 50]. The default DAPT length for patients with ACS treated with coronary stenting should be 12 months, while it may be fair to cut it to 6 months in patients with a high bleeding risk or to extend it to more than 12 months in certain cases. These choices should be made after a thorough assessment of the patients' bleeding and ischemia risks. Although some criteria can aid in the identification of patients who will benefit the most, the requirement to validate surgical tools in clinical practice is well understood. This is especially essential if the DAPT is extended beyond 1 year. A longer dual antiplatelet duration may be considered for patients with this indication who have tolerated this length of DAPT without bleeding problems. In this sense, ticagrelor 60 mg twice daily is advised for patients with a history of myocardial infarction and a high ischemia risk.

4.4 DAPT immediately after transient ischemic attack (TIA) or minor stroke

According to recent *BMJ Rapid Recommendations*, patients with a mild ischemic stroke or a high-risk transient ischemic attack (TIA) should begin dual antiplatelet medication with aspirin and clopidogrel as soon as feasible after the incident, preferably within 24 hours [51]. Dual therapy is favored over aspirin alone, according to the guidelines, because there is a lower risk of recurrent stroke and functional disability with dual therapy. In addition, the guideline committee strongly recommends a shorter term of dual therapy (10–21 days, rather than 22–90 days). Most patients, however, should continue to take a single antiplatelet drug, such as aspirin, continuously. Patients with TIA or mild stroke may benefit from antiplatelet treatment with aspirin and clopidogrel. DAPT with clopidogrel and aspirin (acetylsalicylic acid) within the first 21 days after the index incident was observed to minimize the incidence of recurrent major ischemic events compared to aspirin alone [51]. The recommendations in this clinical practice guideline are based on a linked systematic review sparked by a randomized controlled trial published in August 2018 in the *New England Journal of Medicine* [52].

5. Management of bleeding associated with the use of DAPT

A higher reduction in thrombotic risk comes at the cost of an increase in significant bleedings, which occur in 1–8% of patients in the first year after starting DAPT [53–55]. Even less severe bleeding has been linked to an increased risk of death through indirect mechanisms such as unplanned hospitalization, the necessity for urgent operations, and the termination of DAPT [56]. Bleeding is reportedly linked to an increased risk of death and is also linked to the recurrence of ischemic events such myocardial infarction (MI) and stroke [57, 58].

5.1 Intracranial bleeding (ICB)

The most significant DAPT-related adverse event is intracranial bleeding (ICB). With recurrence rates of more than 15% and 3%, respectively, ICB is classed as lobar (affecting the cerebral cortex and underlying white matter) or deep (affecting the basal ganglia, thalamus, and brainstem). Antiplatelet therapy on admission was linked with a greater 24-hour in-hospital [59] and 3-month death rate compared to naive patients in a recent study on patients with ICB [60].

Patients with ICB should be observed and managed in an intensive care unit or a dedicated stroke unit with a high level of skill in the acute environment. All the anticoagulant and antiplatelet medications should be stopped immediately.

5.2 Gastrointestinal bleeding

GI hemorrhage is the most prevalent significant DAPT-related bleeding event following PCI [61, 62].

Owing to its direct suppression of cyclooxygenase-1, aspirin promotes GI bleeding by lowering the endothelium protective action of prostaglandins. P2Y12 inhibitors are thought to affect ulcer healing through limiting platelet aggregation, angiogenesis, and endothelial proliferation rather than being directly ulcerogenic. When compared to clopidogrel, ticagrelor and prasugrel have been linked to a greater incidence of GI bleeding [61].

Owing to its insidious nature, GI bleeding in patients with recent ACS and/or PCI poses a significant treatment challenge. The need to achieve hemostasis frequently necessitates the early termination of antithrombotic therapy. Furthermore, acute bleeding causes platelet activation, and the formation of a prothrombotic environment could explain why patients with GI bleeding who get DAPT after ACS have a higher risk of ischemic stroke [63].

Proton pump inhibitors (PPIs) should be prescribed alongside antiplatelet medication since gastrointestinal (GI) bleeding is the most prevalent major bleeding event [64]. PPIs are only recommended by the ACC/AHA for individuals who are at risk of bleeding (previous GI bleeding, advanced age, and concurrent use of warfarin, steroids, or nonsteroidal anti-inflammatory medicines); however, the ESC supports PPIs for all DAPT patients [7]. The disparity in recommendations stems from different interpretations of a big clinical research that found a pharmacokinetic interaction between clopidogrel and omeprazole, but no effect on cardiovascular events. Given the known cytochrome pharmacokinetic interaction, it is best to avoid co-prescribing clopidogrel with omeprazole/esomeprazole if at all possible [65]. However, there is no known interaction between PPIs and prasugrel.

5.3 Role of tranexamic acid (TXA) in management of DAPT induced bleeding

Antiplatelet drugs commonly block glycoprotein receptors in ACS because they are required for platelet aggregation. Tranexamic acid (TXA) has been demonstrated to be an effective drug for reduce antiplatelet-related bleeding in a number of clinical scenarios, including trauma, and has a good safety profile [66]. TXA has specifically been shown to increase in vitro platelet activity among coronary artery bypass graft (CABG) patients taking antiplatelet medication as well as demonstrating a reduction in operational blood loss [67]. By enhancing platelet function, TXA can be regarded a potential strategy for reducing bleeding problems associated with antiplatelet monotherapy or DAPT.

5.4 Role of platelet infusions in the management of DAPT-induced bleeding

Platelet concentrates (PCs) are sometimes infused to patients with ICH who are on antiplatelet medications to enhance primary hemostasis before neurosurgery. Platelet concentrates (PCs) are frequently given to patients on APT who develop ICH to overcome platelet inhibition induced by antiplatelet medications [68]. Preoperative transfusion of at least two PCs can enhance primary hemostasis in individuals who require decompression neurosurgery owing to ICH while on APT. Rebleeding could still be a concern especially in individuals with chronic ICH and those using P2Y12 inhibitors. Other options can be explored in the control of bleeding in patients on antiplatelet agents especially DAPT. The options include prothrombin complex concentrates [69] and fresh frozen plasma [70] although they are mostly used for bleeding associated with vitamin K antagonists and direct oral anticoagulants.

6. Conclusion

Antiplatelet agents have been widely utilized in patients with acute coronary syndrome for decades and are increasingly valued for their antithrombotic as well as anti-inflammatory characteristics. DAPT has been shown to be effective in improving the clinical outcomes of patients with ACS or PCI but is associated with high bleeding risk. Recent guidelines have been proposed not only to help reduce the tendency of bleeding in DAPT patients but also to ultimately improve patient overall quality of life.

Acknowledgements

The authors wish to thank the Provost, College of Pharmacy, Afe Babalola University, Professor Femi Oyewo and other lecturers for their support and outstanding encouragement during the course of writing this manuscript.

Conflict of interest

The authors declare no conflict of interest.

Author details

Edidiong Orok[1]*, Funmilayo Adeniyi[2] and Oluwole Akawa[3]

1 Department of Clinical Pharmacy and Public Health, Afe Babalola University, Ado-Ekiti, Nigeria

2 Department of Pharmacology and Toxicology, Afe Babalola University, Ado-Ekiti, Nigeria

3 Department of Pharmaceutical and Medicinal Chemistry, Afe Babalola University, Ado-Ekiti, Nigeria

*Address all correspondence to: pharmorok@gmail.com

References

[1] ISTH Steering Committee for World Thrombosis Day. Thrombosis: A major contributor to the global disease burden. Journal of Thrombosis and Haemostasis. 2014;**12**:1580-1590

[2] White GC, Marder VJ, Schulman S, Aird WC, Bennett JS. Overview of basic coagulation and fibrinolysis. In: Marder VJ, Aird WC, Bennett JS, Schulman S, White GC, editors. Hemostasis and Thrombosis. Basic Principles and Clinical Practice. Philadelphia, PA: Lippincott Williams & Wilkins; 2013. pp. 103-109

[3] Centers for Disease Control and Prevention: About underlying cause of death, 1999-2019. 2018. Available from: https://wonder.cdc.gov/ucd-icd10.html [Accessed: April 12, 2022]

[4] Benjamin E, Muntner P, Alonso A, et al. Heart disease and stroke statistics-2019 update: A report from the American Heart Association. Circulation. 2019;**139**:e56-e528. DOI: 10.1161/CIR.0000000000000659

[5] Chan N, Eikelboom J, Weitz J. Evolving treatments for arterial and venous thrombosis: Role of the direct oral anticoagulants. Circulation Research. 2016;**118**:1409-1424. DOI: 10.1161/CIRCRESAHA.116.306925

[6] Patrono C, Morais J, Baigent C, et al. Antiplatelet agents for the treatment and prevention of coronary atherothrombosis. Journal of the American College of Cardiology. 2017;**70**:1760-1776. DOI: 10.1016/j.jacc.2017.08.037

[7] Valgimigli M, Bueno H, Byrne R, et al. 2017 ESC focused update on dual antiplatelet therapy in coronary artery disease developed in collaboration with EACTS: The task force for dual antiplatelet therapy in coronary artery disease of the European Society of Cardiology (ESC) and of the European Association for Cardio-Thoracic Surgery (EACTS). European Heart Journal. 2018;**39**:213-260. DOI: 10.1093/eurheartj/ehx419

[8] Powers W, Rabinstein A, Ackerson T, et al. Guidelines for the early Management of Patients with Acute Ischemic Stroke: 2019 update to the 2018 guidelines for the early Management of Acute Ischemic Stroke: A guideline for healthcare professionals from the American Heart Association/American Stroke Association. Stroke. 2019;**50**(12):e344-e418. DOI: 10.1161/str.0000000000000211

[9] Kim J, Park M, Choi K, et al. Comparative effectiveness of dual antiplatelet therapy with aspirin and Clopidogrel versus aspirin monotherapy in acute, nonminor stroke: A Nationwide, Multicenter registry-based study. Stroke. 2019;**50**(11):3147-3155

[10] Bhatia K, Jain V, Aggarwal D, et al. Dual antiplatelet therapy versus aspirin in patients with stroke or transient ischemic attack: Meta-analysis of randomized controlled trials. Stroke. 2021;**21**:217-223

[11] Ducrocq G, Amarenco P, Labreuche J, et al. A history of stroke/transient ischemic attack indicates high risks of cardiovascular event and hemorrhagic stroke in patients with coronary artery disease. Circulation. 2013;**127**(6):730-738. DOI: 10.1161/CIRCULATIONAHA.112.141572

[12] Thompson B, Béjot Y, Caso V, et al. Prior antiplatelet therapy and outcome

following intracerebral hemorrhage: A systematic review. Neurology. 2010;**75**(15):1333-1342. DOI: 10.1212/WNL.0b013e3181f735e5

[13] Khan N, Siddiqui F, Goldstein J, et al. Association between previous use of antiplatelet therapy and intracerebral Hemorrhage outcomes. Stroke. 2017;**48**(7):1810-1817. DOI: 10.1161/STROKEAHA.117.016290

[14] Cadavid A. Aspirin: The mechanism of action revisited in the context of pregnancy complications. Frontiers in Immunology. 2017;**8**:261. DOI: 10.3389/fimmu.2017.00261

[15] Tóth L, Muszbek L, Komáromi I. Mechanism of the irreversible inhibition of human cyclooxygenase-1 by aspirin as predicted by QM/MM calculations. Journal of Molecular Graphics & Modelling. 2013;**40**:99-109. DOI: 10.1016/j.jmgm.2012.12.013

[16] Jourdi G, Lordkipanidzé M, Philippe A, Bachelot-Loza C, Gaussem P. Current and novel antiplatelet therapies for the treatment of cardiovascular diseases. International journal of molecular sciences. 2021;**22**(23):13079. DOI: 10.3390/ijms222313079

[17] Van U, Houtenbos I, Griffioen-Keijzer A, et al. Guidelines for mono, double and triple antithrombotic therapy. Postgraduate Medical Journal. 2021;**97**:730-737

[18] Farid N, Smith R, Gillespie T, et al. The disposition of prasugrel, a novel thienopyridine, in humans. Drug Metabolism and Disposition. 2007;**35**: 1096-1004. DOI: 10.1124/dmd.106.014522

[19] Erlinge D, Varenhorst C, Braun O, et al. Patients with poor responsiveness to thienopyridine treatment or with diabetes have lower levels of circulating active metabolite, but their platelets respond normally to active metabolite added ex vivo. Journal of the American College of Cardiology. 2008;**52**:1968-1977. DOI: 10.1016/j.jacc.2008.07.068

[20] Wallentin L. P2Y(12) inhibitors: Differences in properties and mechanisms of action and potential consequences for clinical use. European Heart Journal. 2009;**30**:1964-1977. DOI: 10.1093/eurheartj/ehp296

[21] Nylander S, Femia E, Scavone M, et al. Ticagrelor inhibits human platelet aggregation via adenosine in addition to P2Y12 antagonism. Journal of Thrombosis and Haemostasis. 2013;**11**:1867-1876. DOI: 10.1111/jth.12360

[22] Norgard NB, James JD. Clopidogrel, prasugrel, or ticagrelor? A practical guide to use of antiplatelet agents in patients with acute coronary syndromes. Postgraduate medicine. 2013;**125**(4):91-102. DOI: 10.3810/pgm.2013.07.2682

[23] Alhazzani A, Venkatachalapathy P, Padhilahouse S, et al. Biomarkers for antiplatelet therapies in acute ischemic stroke: A clinical review. Frontiers in Neurology. 2021;**12**:667234. DOI: 10.3389/fneur.2021.667234

[24] Capodanno D, Huber K, Mehran R, et al. Management of antithrombotic therapy in atrial fibrillation patients undergoing PCI: JACC state-of-the-art review. Journal of the American College of Cardiology. 2019;**74**:83-99. DOI: 10.1016/j.jacc.2019.05.016

[25] Gibson C, Mehran R, Bode C, et al. Prevention of bleeding in patients with atrial fibrillation undergoing PCI. The New England Journal of Medicine. 2016;**375**:2423-2434. DOI: 10.1056/NEJMoa1611594

[26] Galli M, Andreotti F, Porto I, Crea F. Intracranial haemorrhages vs. stent thromboses with direct oral anticoagulant plus single antiplatelet agent or triple antithrombotic therapy: A meta-analysis of randomized trials in atrial fibrillation and percutaneous coronary intervention/acute coronary syndrome patients. Europace. 2020;**22**:538-546. DOI: 10.1093/europace/euz345

[27] Steg P, Bhatt D, Simon T, Fox K, Mehta S, Harrington R. Ticagrelor in patients with stable coronary disease and diabetes. The New England Journal of Medicine. 2019;**381**:1309-1320. DOI: 10.1056/NEJMoa1908077

[28] Angiolillo D, Bhatt D, Cannon C, Eikelboom J, Gibson C, Goodman S. Antithrombotic therapy in patients with atrial fibrillation treated with Oral anticoagulation undergoing percutaneous coronary intervention: A north American perspective: 2021 update. Circulation. 2021;**143**(6):583-596. DOI: 10.1161/CIRCULATIONAHA.120.050438

[29] Levine G, Bates E, Bittl J, Brindis R, Fihn S, Fleisher L. 2016 ACC/AHA guideline focused update on duration of dual antiplatelet therapy in patients with coronary artery disease: A report of the American College of Cardiology/American Heart Association task force on clinical practice guidelines. Journal of the American College of Cardiology. 2016;**68**:1082-1115. DOI: 10.1016/j.jacc.2016.03.513

[30] Kimura K, Kimura T, Ishihara M, Nakagawa Y, Nakao K, Miyauchi K. JCS 2018 guideline on diagnosis and treatment of acute coronary syndrome. Circulation Journal. 2019;**83**:1085-1196. DOI: 10.1253/circj.CJ-19-0133

[31] Muscente F, Tautermann G, De Caterina R. Oral anticoagulants for atrial fibrillation and acute coronary syndrome with or without stenting. J cardiovasc med (Hagerstown, Md.). 2018;**19**(1):40-45. DOI: 10.2459/JCM.0000000000000597

[32] Lip G, Collet J, Haude M, Byrne R, Chung E, Fauchier L. 2018 joint European consensus document on the management of antithrombotic therapy in atrial fibrillation patients presenting with acute coronary syndrome and/or undergoing percutaneous cardiovascular interventions: A joint consensus document of the European heart rhythm association (EHRA), European Society of Cardiology Working Group on thrombosis, European Association of Percutaneous Cardiovascular Interventions (EAPCI), and European Association of Acute Cardiac Care (ACCA) endorsed by the Heart Rhythm Society (HRS), Asia-Pacific Heart Rhythm Society (APHRS), Latin America Heart Rhythm Society (LAHRS), and cardiac arrhythmia Society of Southern Africa (CASSA). European Society of Cardiology. 2019;**21**:192-193. DOI: 10.1093/europace/euy174

[33] Saito Y, Kobayashi Y. Update on antithrombotic therapy after percutaneous coronary intervention. Internal Medicine. 2020;**59**:311-321. DOI: 10.2169/internalmedicine.3685-19

[34] Ku J, Taslimi S, Zuccato J, Pasarikovski C, Nasr N, Chechik O. Peri-operative outcomes of carotid endarterectomy are not improved on dual antiplatelet therapy vs. aspirin monotherapy: A systematic review and Meta-analysis. European Journal of Vascular and Endovascular Surgery. 2022;**21**:1030-1033. DOI: 10.1016/j.ejvs.2021.12.037

[35] Neumann F, Sousa-Uva M, Ahlsson A, Alfonso F, Banning A, Benedetto U. 2018 ESC/EACTS

Guidelines on myocardial revascularization. European Heart Journal. 2019;**40**:87-165. DOI: 10.1093/eurheartj/ehy394

[36] Li Z, Xiong Y, Gu H, Fisher M, Xian Y, Johnston S. P2Y12 inhibitors plus aspirin versus aspirin alone in patients with minor stroke or high-risk transient ischemic attack. Stroke. 2021;**52**(7):2250-2257. DOI: 10.1161/STROKEAHA.120.033040

[37] Pomero F, Galli E, Bellesini M, Maroni L, Squizzato A. P2Y12 inhibitors plus aspirin for acute treatment and secondary prevention in minor stroke and high-risk transient ischemic attack: A systematic review and meta-analysis. European Journal of Internal Medicine. 2022;**22**:106-109. DOI: 10.1016/j.ejim.2022.03.017

[38] Kourti O, Konstantas O, Farmakis I, Zafeiropoulos S, Psarakis G, Vrana E. Potent P2Y12 inhibitors versus clopidogrel to predict adherence to antiplatelet therapy after an acute coronary syndrome: Insights from IDEAL-LDL. Reviews in Cardiovascular Medicine. 2022;**23**(3):81. DOI: 10.31083/j.rcm2303081

[39] Kleindorfer D, Towfighi A, Chaturvedi S, Cockroft K, Gutierrez J, Lombardi-Hill D. 2021 guideline for the prevention of stroke in patients with stroke and transient ischemic attack: A guideline from the American Heart Association/American Stroke Association. Stroke. 2021;**52**:364-467. DOI: 10.1161/STR.0000000000000375

[40] Gerhard-Herman M, Gornik H, Barrett C, Barshes N, Corriere M, Drachman D. 2016 AHA/ACC guideline on the Management of Patients with Lower Extremity Peripheral Artery Disease: Executive summary: A report of the American College of Cardiology/American Heart Association task force on clinical practice guidelines. Journal of the American College of Cardiology. 2017;**69**:1465-1508. DOI: 10.1016/j.jacc.2016.11.008

[41] Hamilos M, Petousis S, Xanthopoulou I, Goudevenos J, Kanakakis J, Sitafidis G. Antiplatelet treatment in diabetic patients with acute coronary syndrome undergoing percutaneous coronary intervention: A GReek AntiPlatElet registry substudy. Coronary Artery Disease. 2018;**29**:53-59. DOI: 10.1097/MCA.0000000000000547

[42] Lee T, D'Souza K, Hameed A, Yao J, Lam S, Chadban S. Comparison of the effect of single vs dual antiplatelet agents on post-operative haemorrhage after renal transplantation: A systematic review and meta-analysis. Transplant Rev (Orlando, Fla.). 2021;**35**(1):100594. DOI: 10.1016/j.trre.2020.100594

[43] Antithrombotic Trialists' (ATT) Collaboration, Baigent C, Blackwell L, Collins R, Emberson J, Godwin J. Aspirin in the primary and secondary prevention of vascular disease: Collaborative meta-analysis of individual participant data from randomised trials. Lancet. 2009;**373**(9678):1849-1860. DOI: 10.1016/S0140-6736(09)60503-1

[44] Reaume K, Regal R, Dorsch M. Indications for dual antiplatelet therapy with aspirin and clopidogrel: Evidence-based recommendations for use. The Annals of Pharmacotherapy. 2008;**42**(4):550-557. DOI: 10.1345/aph.1K433

[45] Bonaa K, Mannsverk J, Wiseth R, et al. Drug-eluting or bare-metal stents for coronary artery disease. The New England Journal of Medicine. 2016;**2016**(375):1242-1252. DOI: 10.1056/NEJMoa1607991

[46] Stefanini G, Behan M, Valgimigli M, Oldroyd K, Leon M. Will

LEADERS-FREE change my practice? A randomized double-blind comparison of the bio freedom™ drug-coated stent vs. the gazelle™ bare metal stent in patients at high bleeding risk using a short (1 month) course of dual antiplatelet therapy. EuroInterv. 2016;**12**(16):798-800. DOI: 10.4244/EIJV12I6A129

[47] Tersalvi G, Biasco L, Cioffi G, Pedrazzini G. Acute coronary syndrome, antiplatelet therapy, and bleeding: A clinical perspective. Journal of Clinical Medicine. 2020;**9**(7):2064. DOI: 10.3390/jcm9072064

[48] Mauri L, Kereiakes D, Yeh R, Driscoll-Shempp P, Cutlip D, Steg P. Twelve or 30 months of dual antiplatelet therapy after drug-eluting stents. The New England Journal of Medicine. 2014;**371**(23):2155-2166. DOI: 10.1056/NEJMoa1409312

[49] Roffi M, Patrono C, Collet J, Mueller C, Valgimigli M, Andreotti F. 2015 ESC guidelines for the management of acute coronary syndromes in patients presenting without persistent ST-segment elevation: Task force for the Management of Acute Coronary Syndromes in patients presenting without persistent ST-segment elevation of the European Society of Cardiology (ESC). European Heart Journal. 2016;**37**:267-315

[50] Ibanez B, James S, Agewall S, Antunes M, Bucciarelli-Ducci C, Bueno H. 2017 ESC guidelines for the management of acute myocardial infarction in patients presenting with ST-segment elevation. European Heart Journal. 2018;**39**:119-177

[51] Hao Q, Tampi M, O'Donnell M, Foroutan F, Siemieniuk R, Guyatt G. Clopidogrel plus aspirin versus aspirin alone for acute minor ischaemic stroke or high risk transient ischaemic attack: Systematic review and meta-analysis. BMJ. 2018;**363**:k5108. DOI: 10.1136/bmj.k5108

[52] Johnston S, Easton J, Farrant M, et al. Clopidogrel and aspirin in acute ischemic stroke and high-risk TIA. The New England Journal of Medicine. 2018;**379**:215-225. DOI: 10.1056/NEJMoa1800410 pmid:29766750

[53] Roe M, Armstrong P, Fox K, et al. Prasugrel versus clopidogrel for acute coronary syndromes without revascularization. The New England Journal of Medicine. 2012;**367**(14):1297-1309. DOI: 10.1056/NEJMoa1205512

[54] Baber U, Sartori S, Aquino M. Use of prasugrel vs clopidogrel and outcomes in patients with acute coronary syndrome undergoing percutaneous coronary intervention in contemporary clinical practice: Results from the PROMETHEUS study. American Heart Journal. 2017;**188**:73-81. DOI: 10.1016/j.ahj.2017.02.013

[55] Park D, Kwon O, Jang J, et al. Clinically significant bleeding with Ticagrelor versus Clopidogrel in Korean patients with acute coronary syndromes intended for invasive management: A randomized clinical trial. Circulation. 2019;**140**(23):1865-1877. DOI: 10.1161/CIRCULATIONAHA.119.041766

[56] Halvorsen S, Storey RF, Rocca B, et al. Management of antithrombotic therapy after bleeding in patients with coronary artery disease and/or atrial fibrillation: Expert consensus paper of the European Society of Cardiology Working Group on thrombosis. Eur. 2017;**38**(19):1455-1462. DOI: 10.1093/eurheartj/ehw454

[57] Palmerini T, Bacchi Reggiani L, Della Riva D, Romanello M, Feres F, Abizaid A. Bleeding-related deaths in relation to the duration of dual-antiplatelet therapy

after coronary stenting. Journal of the American College of Cardiology. 2017;**69**(16):2011-2022. DOI: 10.1016/j.jacc.2017.02.029

[58] Valgimigli M, Costa F, Lokhnygina Y, Clare R, Wallentin L, Moliterno D. Trade-off of myocardial infarction vs. bleeding types on mortality after acute coronary syndrome: Lessons from the thrombin receptor antagonist for clinical event reduction in acute coronary syndrome (TRACER) randomized trial. Eur. 2017;**38**(11):804-810. DOI: 10.1093/eurheartj/ehw525

[59] Franco L, Paciaroni M, Enrico M, Scoditti U, Guideri F, Chiti A. Mortality in patients with intracerebral hemorrhage associated with antiplatelet agents, oral anticoagulants or no antithrombotic therapy. European Journal of Internal Medicine. 2020;**75**:35-43. DOI: 10.1016/j.ejim.2019.12.016

[60] Roquer J, Vivanco Hidalgo R, Ois A, Rodríguez Campello A, Cuadrado GE. Antithrombotic pretreatment increases very-early mortality in primary intracerebral hemorrhage. Neurology. 2017;**88**(9):885-891. DOI: 10.1212/WNL.0000000000003659

[61] Becker R, Bassand J, Budaj A, et al. Bleeding complications with the P2Y12 receptor antagonists clopidogrel and ticagrelor in the PLATelet inhibition and patient outcomes (PLATO) trial. Eur. 2011;**32**:2933-2944

[62] Généreux P, Giustino G, Witzenbichler B, et al. Incidence, predictors, and impact of post-discharge bleeding after percutaneous coronary intervention. Journal of the American College of Cardiology. 2015;**66**:1036-1045

[63] Nikolsky E, Stone G, Kirtane A, et al. Gastrointestinal bleeding in patients with acute coronary syndromes: Incidence, predictors, and clinical implications: Analysis from the ACUITY (acute catheterization and urgent intervention triage strategy) trial. Journal of the American College of Cardiology. 2009;**54**(14):1293-1302. DOI: 10.1016/j.jacc.2009.07.019

[64] Agewall S, Cattaneo M, Collet J, et al. Expert position paper on the use of proton pump inhibitors in patients with cardiovascular disease and antithrombotic therapy. Eur. 2013;**34**(23):1708-713b. DOI: 10.1093/eurheartj/eht042

[65] Floyd C, Passacquale G, Ferro A. Comparative pharmacokinetics and pharmacodynamics of platelet adenosine diphosphate receptor antagonists and their clinical implications. Clinical Pharmacokinetics. 2012;**51**(7):429-442. DOI: 10.2165/11630740-000000000-00000

[66] Fischer K, Awudi E, Varon J, Surani S. Role of tranexamic acid in the clinical setting. Cureus. 2020;**12**:8221. DOI: 10.7759/cureus.8221\

[67] Banihashem N, Khorasani M, Vaffai H, et al. The effect of low- dose tranexamic acid on postoperative blood loss in patients treated with clopidogrel and aspirin. Caspian Journal of Internal Medicine. 2019;**10**:156-161. DOI: 10.22088/cjim.10.2.156

[68] Fogarty P. Intracranial haemorrhage: Therapeutic interventions and anaesthetic management. British Journal of Anaesthesia. 2014;**113**(Suppl 2):17-25

[69] Johansen M, Wikkelsø A, Lunde J, Wetterslev J, Afshari A. Prothrombin complex concentrate for reversal of vitamin K antagonist treatment in bleeding and non-bleeding patients. Cochrane Database of Systematic Reviews. 2015;**2015**(7):CD010555. DOI: 10.1002/14651858.CD010555.pub2

[70] Straus S, Haxhibeqiri-Karabdic I, Grabovica SG, Granov N. A difference in bleeding and use of blood and blood products in patients who were preoperatively on aspirin or dual antiplatelet therapy before coronary artery bypass grafting. Med Arch. 2018;**72**(1):31-35. DOI: 10.5455/medarh.2018.72.31-35

Chapter 6

Recent Advances in Catheter Ablation for Atrial Fibrillation and Non-pharmacological Stroke Prevention

Nayanjyoti Kaushik, James Arter Chapman, Andrew Gillaspie, Stephen Ackerman, Peter Gallagher, Deobrat Mallick and Steven J. Bailin

Abstract

Atrial Fibrillation is a common arrhythmia affecting 6 million people in the United States and 33 million people worldwide, associated with significant morbidity. Whereas restoration and maintenance of sinus rhythm can translate into clinical benefit, early intervention in course of the disease can influence success and efficacy of intervention has been speculative and uncertain over past decade despite several literature and scientific studies. During past three decades catheter and surgical ablation of AF have evolved from an investigational status to a widely offerred definitive treatment now. With recent advances in mapping technology, ablation energy delivery, better understanding of pathogenesis and mechanism of AF there has been a paradigm shift in clinical decision making, patient selection, patient-physician discussion about various rhythm control strategy due to an ever improving safety and efficacy of the procedure. In this chapter we will briefly review the landmark clinical trials that has changed the outlook towards rhythm control strategy beginning from early trials such as AFFIRM, telling us rhythm control was no better than rate control to recent studies and EAST AFNET, which showed benefits of rhythm control. We will discuss differences in ablation strategy, safety and efficacy between paroxysmal AF vs. Persistent/ Longstanding Persistent AF from a trigger and substrate view and pulmonary vein and non pulmonary vein targets for ablation. We will also elaborate on different energy sources for ablation such as Radiofrequency (RF), Cryoablation, newer ablation techniques such as Vein of Marshall alcohol ablation, High Power short duration ablation, Pulsed Field Ablation, Surgical ablation and Hybrid Convergent Ablation etc. Since this chapter is mostly intended towards diagnosis and management of AF in twenty-first century, authors have restricted mainly to recent developments only and purposefully have not expanded on already established preexisting knowledge about topics such as pharmacological rhythm control, rate control, Atrio-Ventricular node ablation with pacemaker implantation, direct current cardio version etc. In conclusion, with recent emerging evidence, importance of rhythm control is being increasingly recognized. Catheter ablation is more commonly performed with improving safety and efficacy. There are newer technology and ablation strategy available and should be offered to patient while discussing a comprehensive management of AF with careful review of risk benefit analysis.

Keywords: catheter ablation, atrial fibrillation, rhythm control, pulmonary vein isolation, pulse field ablation, vein of marshal, cardioneural ablation, ganglionic plexi, high power short duration, cryoablation, radiofrequency ablation, left atrial appendage occlusion, watchman, stroke prevention

1. Introduction

Atrial Fibrillation is well known to cause not only substantial morbidity including stroke, congestive heart failure, and late cognitive impairment, dementia [1, 2] but is also associated with reduced survival. In subjects from the original cohort of the Framingham Heart Study, AF was associated with a 1.5- to 1.9-fold mortality risk after adjustment for the preexisting cardiovascular conditions with which AF was related [3]. This common cardiac arrhythmia, that increases in prevalence with advancing age, poses a perplexing treatment situation to clinicians as symptomatology varies in a wide spectrum. Symptoms can be asymptomatic in one extreme to frequent hospitalizations, hemodynamic abnormalities, and even thromboembolic events related to AF [4] which increase morbidity and mortality in the other. Despite numerous trials and scientific data it is inconclusive whereas restoration and maintenance of sinus rhythm is associated with clinically meaningful benefits, preferred strategy of rhythm control e.g. catheter ablation vs. anti arrhythmic drugs etc.

2. Brief literature review of landmark trials on benefits of rhythm control

Initial RCTs [5, 6] failed to show superiority of rhythm control on mortality [4], however maintenance of sinus rhythm did show improvement in quality of life and exercise capacity [7, 8]. These particular studies did not include patients with catheter ablation and most patients underwent rhythm control with repeated cardioversions and Antiarrhythmic drugs. Bunch et al. [9] published AF ablation patients have a significantly lower risk of death, stroke, and dementia in comparison to AF patients without ablation. Various experimental studies [10] and scientific position papers [11, 12] have indicated that early intervention with a rhythm-control strategy to prevent progression of AF may be beneficial [4] which eluded to the fact that "AF begets AF" due to electrical and structural myocardial left atrial remodeling. Subsequently, several RCTs have tested the strategy of catheter ablation vs. medical management as discussed below.

MANTRA PAF [13] was one of the initial trials that enrolled 294 patients (June 2005 through 2009) with symptomatic Paroxysmal Atrial Fibrillation (PAF) with no history of antiarrhythmic drug use. These patients were treated with either radiofrequency catheter ablation (146 patients) or therapy with Class IC or Class III antiarrhythmic agents (148 patients) [13]. This trial found no significant difference in cumulative AF burden between both treatment groups over a follow up of 24 months but the burden of symptomatic atrial fibrillation and any atrial fibrillation was significantly lower in the ablation group than in the drug-therapy group. These findings suggested that the efficacy of catheter ablation may be more durable than that of currently available antiarrhythmic drugs. There was no difference in quality of life between both treatment arms, but a perception of more improvement in physical well-being was seen in the ablation group which authors admitted that this may be attributable in part to a placebo effect. There were 36% of patients who were initially assigned to AAD arm who subsequently required ablation for recurrent atrial fibrillation, a finding signaling that though an initial rhythm control strategy with AAD may be initiated, a minority of such patients may subsequently require catheter ablation for adequate rhythm control. A major limitation of this trial was definition of goal of ablation for atrial fibrillation. At the time of the study, this was defined as elimination of complex high frequency electrograms inside encircled areas around the Pulmonary Veins (PV), but with rapid development of ablation techniques, this end point was no longer valid. A general agreement on end point of ablation is considered complete electrical isolation of pulmonary veins. A change in ablation strategy based on this end point may have potentially changed the outcome of the study.

RAAFT 2 [14]. was another contemporary RCT to MANTRA PAF enrolling 127 patients with symptomatic PAF from Europe and North America between July 2006 to January 2010 and then patients were followed up for 2 years till 2012. Patients were randomized to ablation vs. anti arrhythmic treatment arms. Ablation was performed with circumferential pulmonary vein isolation with demonstration of entrance block into pulmonary vein, with additional ablation such as linear lines in Left Atrium (LA), ganglionic plexi, targeting complex fractionated electrogram, superior vena cava (SVC) isolation, cavotricuspid isthmus (CTI) ablation all at the investigator's discretion [14]. With change in ablation goal when compared to MANTRA PAF, RAAFT 2 trial demonstrated catheter ablation resulted in significantly lower rate of recurrent atrial tachyarrhythmia at 2 years, and reduced the frequency of repeated episodes of AF and thus improvement in quality of life however, recurrence was documented in approximately 50% of patients. Ablation extends the time free of both symptomatic and asymptomatic AF and significantly reduced the recurrence of repeated episodes, potentially having an effect on AF progression [14]. This study was limited by small sample size, and findings restricted to mostly young people with PAF. So authors suggested that when offering ablation as a therapeutic option to patients with paroxysmal AF naive to antiarrhythmic drugs, the risks and benefits need to be discussed and treatment strategy individually recommended.

Rhythm control vs. rate control for AF in patients with heart failure (HF) were studied in multiple studies. In a multi center RCT [15], 1376 patients who had congestive heart failure with EF ≤ 35% were enrolled. Maintenance of sinus rhythm with Antiarrhythmic drugs did not reduce the rate of death from cardiovascular causes, as compared with a rate-control strategy. Role of catheter ablation was however not studied in this RCT. Significant proportion of patients do not tolerate anti arrhythmic drugs due to various side effects, is not responsive to AAD, or has difficulty in medication adherence or compliance. Catheter ablation is a suitable alternative for rhythm control. There have been several studies that has shown positive effect of ablation in AF and CHF patients [16–20]. CASTLE AF was a landmark large multi center open labeled randomized control trial [21] where 398 patients were enrolled with symptomatic Paroxysmal or Persistent AF who failed, had unacceptable side effects, or had an unwillingness to take antiarrhythmic drugs. These patients also had New York Heart Association (NYHA) Class II, III, or IV heart failure and a left ventricular ejection fraction (LVEF) of 35% or less. As compared to multiple previous trials showing benefit of catheter ablation [16–20], this was the first trial that tested the effectiveness of catheter ablation in improving rates of hard primary end points such as death or the progression of heart failure. Primary end point which was a composite of death from any cause and lower rates of hospital admission for heart failure was significantly fewer in the ablation group. In addition there were other secondary outcomes seen such as increase in LVEF and reduction in AF burden.

CABANA trial [1] (published in 2019) was a landmark trial that enrolled 2204 symptomatic AF patients (paroxysmal, persistent and long persistent) from 126 centers over 10 countries and tested catheter ablation vs. medical management with antiarrhythmic and/or rate control medications. Catheter ablation did not significantly reduce the primary composite end point of death, disabling stroke, serious bleeding, or cardiac arrest, but secondary end point of mortality or CV hospitalization showed a significant 17% relative lower event rate for the catheter ablation group [1]. Post 90 day blanking period, patients were monitored for time to first AF recurrence defined as AF/AFl/AT for ≥30 s. Catheter ablation was associated with a lower AF recurrence rate than drug therapy (50% vs. 69% at 3 years post blanking follow-up). Another significant observation in this study was low rate of procedure related complication seen in catheter ablation group indicating that ablation is feasible. The trial had several limitations [1] such as higher rate of patient withdrawal in drug therapy group, catheter ablation and drug therapy may have changed over the long course of the trial, small percentage of patients may have received only rate control drugs. Comparisons of the intention to treat (ITT) results with the treatment received and per-protocol analyses suggest that the combined effect of crossovers and withdrawals reduced the estimated treatment effect and the precision of the effect size estimates as assessed by ITT. Additionally, potential introduction of bias due to unblinded site adjudication of cause of hospitalization etc. might have affected the results of the study. Authors concluded that the estimated treatment effect of catheter ablation was affected by lower-than-expected event rates and treatment crossovers, which should be considered in interpreting the results of the trial.

With initial belief that rhythm control strategy is not superior over rate control, based on AFFIRM study published in early first decade of twenty-first century, we have witnessed through several trials discussed above, the evolution of scientific evidence demonstrating efficacy of ablation strategy in improving quality of life, improvement of heart failure symptoms, improvement of exercise tolerance, survival benefits, reduce hospitalization etc. A monumental trial that brought a paradigm shift is EAST AFNET 4 [22]. This study was published in 2020 and sought to compare early rhythm control vs. usual care. This was a multi center randomized trial that enrolled over 2700 patients from 135 sites in 11 countries. Early rhythm control required antiarrhythmic drugs or atrial fibrillation ablation, as well as cardioversion of persistent atrial fibrillation, to be initiated early after randomization. Usual care arm patients were initially treated with only rate control therapy and rhythm-control therapy was used only to mitigate uncontrolled atrial fibrillation–related symptoms during adequate rate-control therapy. The trial was stopped for efficacy at the third interim analysis after a median of 5.1 years of follow-up per patient. The first primary outcome was a composite of death from cardiovascular causes, stroke (either ischemic or hemorrhagic), or hospitalization with worsening of heart failure or acute coronary syndrome [22]. First primary outcome event was found to have occurred less often in patients assigned to early rhythm control than in patients assigned to usual care achieving a conclusion that early rhythm control was beneficial that was associated with lower risk of adverse cardiovascular outcomes [22]. The results of this study was different from previously published studies comparing rhythm vs. rate control because of incorporation of catheter ablation which is a powerful tool for restoring sinus rhythm.

Another recent study, STOP-AF First [23] was published in 2021 which compared the efficacy of cryoboalloon ablation over AAD in patients with symptomatic paroxysmal AF. Cryoballoon ablation as initial therapy was superior to drug therapy for the prevention of atrial arrhythmia recurrence in patients with paroxysmal atrial fibrillation with low procedure related adverse events.

There are three modes for rhythm control: Electrical (direct current cardioversion), Pharmacological (Antiarrhythmic mediation) and catheter ablation. With the scope of this chapter we will focus more on evolution and rapid advent of catheter ablation strategy over past few years (**Figure 1**).

Current AHA/ACC/HRS Atrial Fibrillation guidelines [4] and 2017 HRS/EHRA/ECAS/APHRS/SOLAECE expert consensus statement on catheter and surgical ablation of atrial fibrillation recommend catheter ablation in patients with symptomatic PAF (COR Class I) who are intolerant or refractory to Class I or Class III AAD, or ablation as initial strategy before trial of AAD (COR Class IIa). In recent 2019 focused update new recommendation have been added as AF catheter ablation may be reasonable in selected patients with symptomatic AF and HF with reduced left ventricular (LV) ejection fraction (HFrEF) to potentially lower mortality rate and reduce hospitalization for HF based on evidence from CASTLE AF data (COR Class IIb, LOE B-R) (**Table 1**) [24].

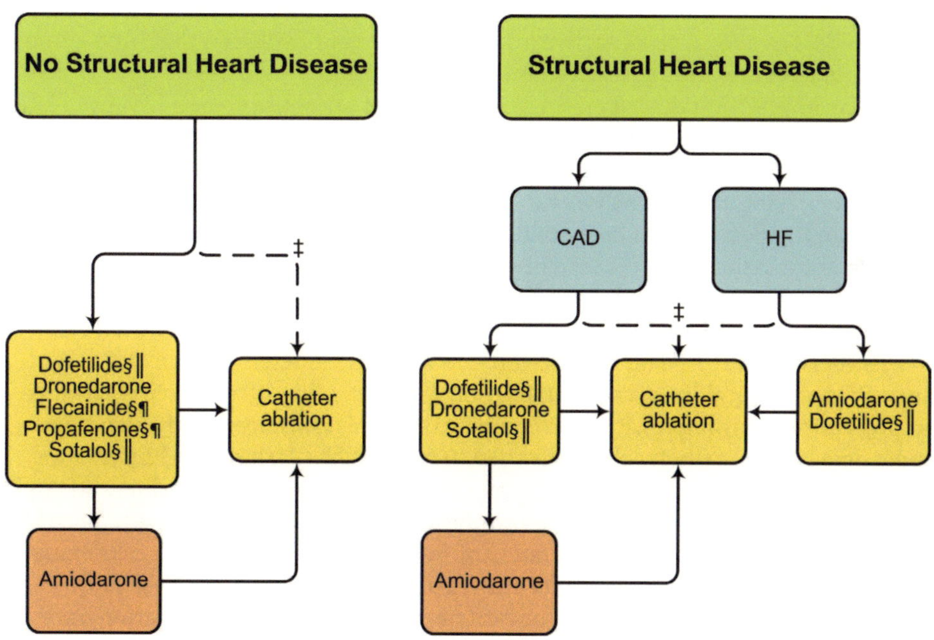

Figure 1.
Strategies for rhythm control in patients with paroxysmal and persistent AF†. *Catheter ablation is only recommended as first-line therapy for patients with paroxysmal AF (Class IIa recommendation). †Drugs are listed alphabetically. ‡Depending on patient preference when performed in experienced centers. §Not recommended with severe LVH (wall thickness > 1.5 cm). ‖Should be used with caution in patients at risk for torsades de pointes ventricular tachycardia. ¶Should be combined with AV nodal blocking agents. AF indicates atrial fibrillation; AV, atrioventricular; CAD, coronary artery disease; HF, heart failure; and LVH, left ventricular hypertrophy. Adopted from [4].*

COR	LOE	Recommendation
Class I	A	Ablation useful in Symptomatic PAF who are refractory/intolerant to at least one Class I/III AAD
Class IIa	B	Ablation reasonable in recurrent symptomatic PAF before trial of Class I/III AAD
Class IIa	A	Ablation reasonable in Persistent symptomatic AF who are refractory/intolerant to at least one Class I/III AAD
Class IIa	B-NR	It is reasonable to offer AF ablation as an alternative to pacemaker implantation in patients with tachy-brady syndrome.
Class IIb	B-R	Ablation reasonable in selected patients with symptomatic AF and HFrEF) to potentially lower mortality rate and reduce hospitalization for HF [24]
Class IIb	B	Ablation reasonable in long standing symptomaticPersistent AF (>12 months) who are refractory/intolerant to at least one Class I/III AAD
Class IIb	B	Ablation reasonable in Persistent symptomatic AF before trial of Class I/III AAD

Table 1.
Professional society guideline recommendations for atrial fibrillation catheter ablation.

3. Catheter ablation of atrial fibrillation

Pathogenesis of AF is incompletely understood. Broadly generalized, there is a trigger that initiate AF and there is a perpetuating factor that sustain the arrhythmia. Usually a PAC or a focal atrial tachycardia triggers atrial fibrillation that further creates a rapid irregular multiple wavelets of depolarization.

Dr. Cox in 1987 first described surgical ablation of atrial fibrillation [25] by creating multiple scars by "cut and sew" technique to create lines of conduction block to prevent atrial reentry and allow sinus impulses to activate the entire atrial myocardium, thereby preserving atrial transport function postoperatively. However, application of the maze III operation has been limited by the morbidity and risk associated with sternotomy-thoracotomy and cardiopulmonary bypass, as well as by limited adoption by cardiothoracic surgeons [26]. Seminal publication by Dr. Michel Haïssaguerre [27] in 1998 that pulmonary vein ectopics are frequent triggers for AF and ablation of these foci can treat AF laid the initial foundation for catheter ablation of AF. With the success of surgical lines, catheter ablation was tried with different curve sheaths but procedure was fraught with high complication rates and exceedingly high fluoroscopic times. Initial catheter ablations tried to target Right Atrium (RA) by creating Intercaval lines along the interatrial septum and Cavotricuspid isthmus line and target Left Atrium (LA) by creating three or four lines. Pappone and Co workers published Circumferential Radiofrequency Ablation of Pulmonary Vein Ostia with electroanatomic guidance is safe and effective in either paroxysmal or permanent AF [28].

Since then, different approachs for catheter ablation for atrial fibrillation have evolved such as segmental ostial PV Isolation, circumferential antral Pulmonary vein isolation (PVI), wide area circumferential LA ablation, catheter Maze (lines to connect the ipsilateral pairs of the PVs and a line to link the left PV encircling lesion to the mitral annulus), complex fractionated electrogram ablation (CFAE), Box lesion sets with linear lines ("floor line" and "roof line") to isolate posterior wall, Left atrial Appendage (LAA) isolation, Superior Vena Cava (SVC) isolation, autonomic ganglionated plexi ablation or Cardioneural ablation, alcohol ablation of vein of Marshal etc. There is no clear consensus about efficacy of one approach over another,

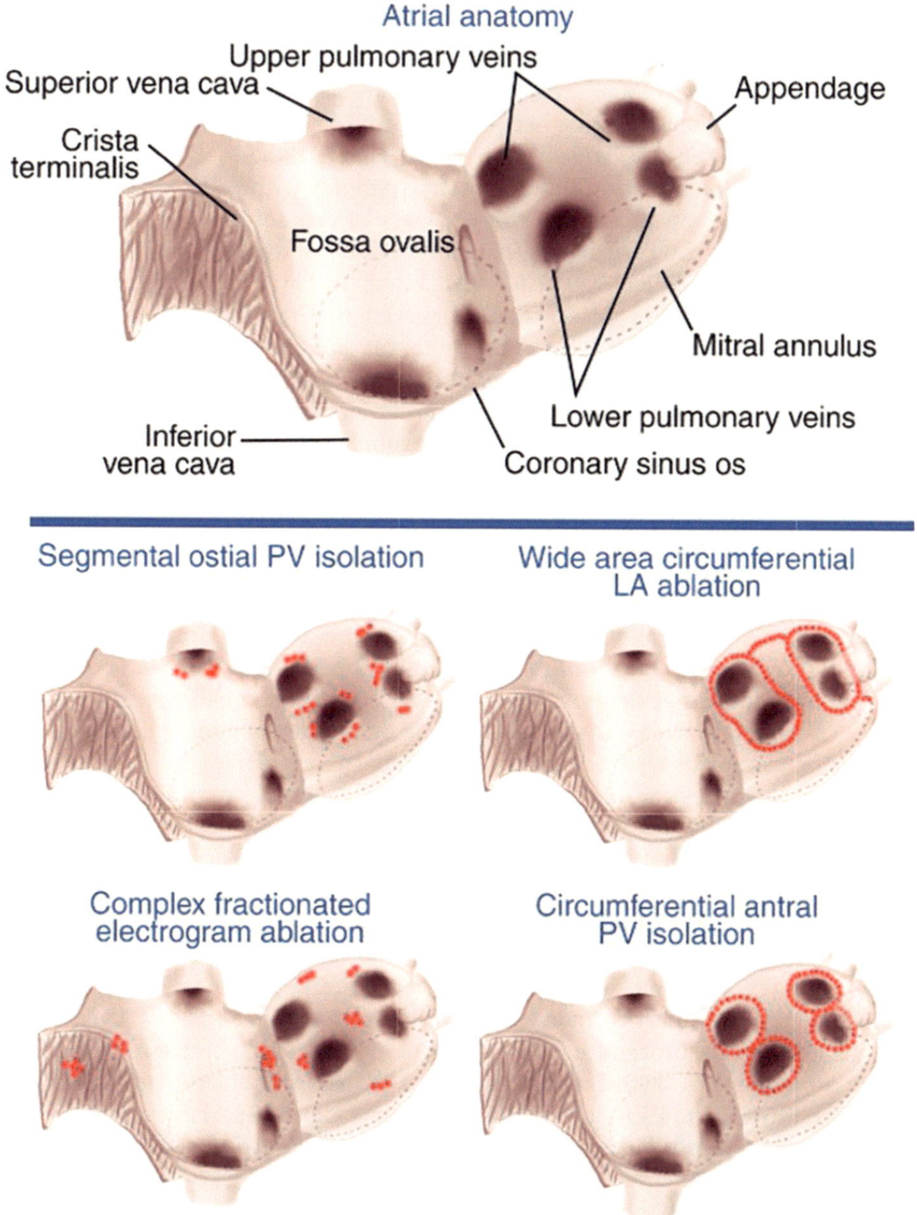

Figure 2.
Schematic diagram of various approaches of catheter ablation shown. Red circles are ablation lesions. Picture adopted from [26].

but approaches often vary between paroxysmal Atrial Fibrillation and persistent Atrial Fibrillation. In PAF targeting the trigger for Atrial Fibrillation with wide antral circumferential ablation of bilateral PVs may prove sufficient in freedom from recurrent AF/AFl/AT. In contrast, patients with persistent Atrial Fibrillation, both trigger and substrate needs to be ablated and ablation may be necessary beyond routine PVI which may include posterior wall isolation or additional linear lines in left atrium depending on operator's discretion (**Figure 2**).

3.1 Substrate based ablation for persistent/long persistent atrial fibrillation: targeting pulmonary and non pulmonary vein triggers

Though PV are most frequent triggers for AF, investigators have shown several non PV triggers, incidence ranging between 3.2% and 47%, especially in Persistent/ Long standing Persistent AF. Triggers have been demonstrated in SVC (common in female patients), LA posterior wall, (common in patients with enlarged LA), Crista terminals, Left atrial appendage, Coronary sinus, Ligament of Marshall, Interatrial septum. Additionally, SVTs such as AVN reentrant tachycardia (AVNRT) and AV reentrant tachycardia (AVRT) can be identified in up to 4% in unselected patients referred for AF ablation and can serve as a triggering mechanism for AF [26]. Previous studies have suggested a benefit to intervention with ablation before drug failure, because a shorter "diagnosis-to-ablation" time is associated with lower rates of arrhythmia recurrence or repeat procedures and fewer hospitalizations [29–31].

STAR AF II [32] was a randomized trial that compared efficacy of three different approaches to catheter ablation of AF in patients with Persistent AF. They randomized patients into three arms: (1) PVI alone (2) PVI with CFAE (3) PVI and Linear ablation lines along the LA roof and Mitral Isthmus. Primary outcome of the study was to see any documented episode of atrial fibrillation lasting longer than 30 s and occurring after the performance of a single ablation procedure, with or without the use of antiarrhythmic medications. Clinical assessments, 12-lead electrocardiograms, and 24-h Holter-monitor recordings were obtained at baseline and at 3, 6, 9, 12, and 18 months after the initial ablation. Study showed no reduction in the rate of recurrent atrial fibrillation when either linear ablation or ablation of complex fractionated electrograms was performed in addition to pulmonary-vein isolation. Recurrence of atrial arrhythmia despite extensive ablation on a substrate based approach with targets beyond PV such as CFAE, linear lines probably created iatrogenic areas of arrhythmogenesis potentially from incomplete ablation of areas with complex electrograms or conduction gaps in linear lines.

A meta-analysis of 113 studies including 18,657 patients examined the impact of ablation approach on outcomes associated with Persistent or Long standing persistent AF [33]. Findings of this meta-analysis supports the findings of the STAR AF II trial, with collated results indicating that a simpler PVI approach (57% success) yields at least equivalent single-procedure results (or potentially better) compared with more complex substrate ablation techniques including PVI + Linear ablation lines (46%), PVI + CFAE (46%), and PVI + Linear ablation lines + CFAE (33%) as currently performed and reported. This study also concluded that the efficacy of a single-AF ablation procedure for Persistent or Long standing persistent AF is 43%; however, can be increased to 69% with the use of multiple procedures and/or anti-arrhythmic drug.

3.2 Left atrial appendage electrical isolation/vein of marshall alcohol ablation

BELIEF trial [34] is an RCT that included 173 patients with long standing persistent atrial fibrillation that were randomized into two arms: (1) Standard ablation arm that comprised of an extended PV antrum ablation plus non-PV trigger ablation (2) standard ablation plus empirical electrical left atrial appendage isolation. Primary end point of the study was freedom from atrial arrhythmia (AF, A Fl, AT) defined as >30 s after initial 12 weeks blanking period while off anti arrhythmic drugs, secondary end points were 12-month post-procedure incidence of stroke, death, and rehospitalization. Trial results showed that in patients with Long standing Persistent

AF, empirical isolation of LAA improved long-term freedom from atria arrhythmia without increasing complications. An important finding to consider however is life long need for uninterrupted anticoagulation in patients who underwent LAA isolation as post procedure lack of proper mechanical function in the LAA may contribute to stroke.

Recently, Alcohol ablation of Vein of Marshall (VoM) has gained significant attention. This method of ethanol infusion into VoM in addition to catheter ablation was investigated in VENUS [35] RCT. 343 patients with Persistent AF were randomized into catheter ablation alone vs. catheter ablation with VoM ethanol infusion. Primary end point was freedom from AF/AT > 30 s without AAD at 6 and 12 months, several secondary endpoints including AF burden, freedom from AF after multiple procedures, perimitral block, and others were studied. VoM is the embryological remnant of left superior vena cava is implicated as AF trigger, parasympathetic and sympathetic innervation contributing to AF, located in the mitral isthmus contributing to perimitral atrial tachycardia. Results of this study concluded that addition of VoM ethanol infusion to catheter ablation increased the likelihood of remaining free of AF or atrial tachycardia at 6 and 12 months. Adverse events were not significantly different between both group: intraprocedural pericardial effusion occurred in two patients in VoM ethanol infusion group (one in ablation only group), subacute pericardial effusion requiring drainage occurred in four patients (two in each group), symptomatic inflammatory pericarditis not requiring drainage occurred in 11 patients in the VoM ethanol infusion group and in 6 in the catheter ablation group. The benefits of VoM ethanol infusion in addition to

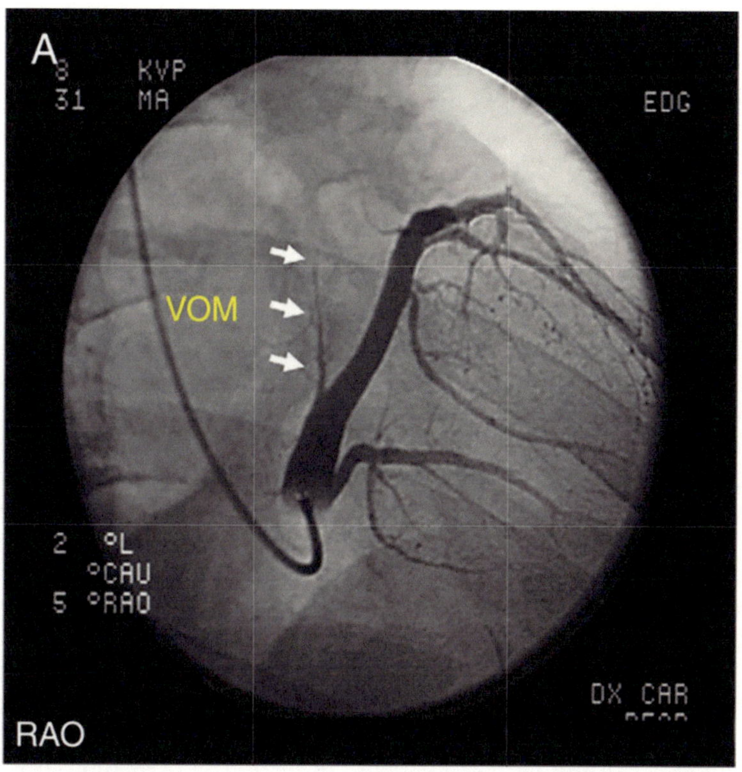

Figure 3.
Coronary sinus venogram showing vein of Marshall. Picture adopted from [26].

	Recommendation	Class	LOE
PVI by catheter ablation	Electrical Isolation of PV during all AF ablation procedure	Class I	A
	Achievment of Isolation requires at a minimum, assessment and demonstration of entrance block into the PV.	Class I	B-R
	Monitoring for 20 min following initial isolation	Class IIa	B-R
	Administration of Adenosine to see if reconnection occurred, demonstration of exit block, pace capture ablation strategy may be considered	Class IIb	B-R B-NR
CTI ablation	If there is history of typical A Fl or inducible during ablation, CTI ablation is recommended	Class I	B-R
Ablation strategies to be considered for use in conjunction with PV isolation	If linear ablation is performed, mapping and pacing maneuvers should be performed to check for line completeness If reproducible focal trigger outside PV ostium that initiates AF are seen, ablation should be considered	Class I Class IIa	C-LD C-LD
	Posterior wall isolation might be considered for initial or repeat ablation of persistent or long- standing persistent AF	Class IIb	C-LD

Table 2.
Professional society recommendations for catheter and surgical ablation strategies and endpoints.

catheter ablation was attributed to elimination of AF trigger, achieving more reliable perimitral block, enhanced atrial denervation (**Figure 3**).

2017 HRS/EHRA/ECAS/APHRS/SOLAECE Expert Consensus Statement on Catheter and Surgical Ablation of Atrial Fibrillation recommends following Atrial fibrillation ablation strategies, techniques, and endpoints (**Table 2**).

3.3 High power short duration (HPSD) ablation

High power short duration (HPSD) ablation strategy is a newer approach in effective lesion formation. Conventionally AF ablation has been performed with low power long duration (LPLD) at 25–35 W power delivery for 30–60 s per lesion. Success of AF ablation is dependent on durability of lesions that in turn is influenced by several variables like catheter stability, orientation of ablation catheter (perpendicular vs. parallel), time duration, effective power and current delivered at catheter tip, transmurality of lesion etc. HPSD (50–80 W power for 5 s) was initially described by Bhaskaran et al. [36] in 2016 as safe and effective as the conventional ablation. Current definition of HPSD varies between power of 50–90 s and time duration of 2–20 s. Based on principles of biophysics of Radiofrequency (RF) ablation, HPSD is believed to cause majority of tissue death via resistive heating and, as a result, theoretical advantages have been proposed, including optimized lesion geometry, reduced collateral tissue damage and increased durability of electrical isolation, in addition to obvious benefits in reduction in procedural duration [37]. Winkle et al. [38] reported very low complication rates with HPSD (45–50 W for 2–10 s) compared to LPLD (35 W for 20 s) in total of 13,974 ablations performed in 10,284 patients, of these, 11,436 ablations performed in the posterior wall. They also found HPSD ablations shorten procedural and total RF times and create more localized and durable lesions. Recently, Very High Power Short

Duration (vHPSD) with 90 W for 4 s with a novel catheter design (THERMOCOOL SMARTTOUCH SF-5D System) was studied in Q DOT FAST trial [39] where 52 patients with PAF underwent ablation with no deaths, stroke, atrioesophageal fistula, pulmonary vein stenosis, or unanticipated adverse device effects. This study showed safety, feasibility and short term efficacy of vHPSD ablation along with substantial reduction in procedural and fluoroscopic time. Currently there is an ongoing prospective clinical trial (HIPAF) comparing two strategies: HPSD-PVI (70 W over 5 s posterior and 7 s anterior) ablation vs. Cryo PVI [40].

3.4 Pulsed Field Ablation (PFA)

So far, RF or Cryo ablation has been the only two available technologies for endocardial ablation of Atrial Fibrillation. In recent years, clinical research on an emerging modality for cardiac ablation has demonstrated significant advantages over existing thermal ablation modalities. Irreversible Electroporation is a non thermal modality with emerging application in the field of cardiology with more selective and effective ablation with minimal surrounding tissue damage. Dr. Steven Mickelsen at University of Iowa developed Pulsed Field Ablation (PFA) system and adapted catheters to deliver pulsed field electricity to the tissue for treating AF with his start up called "IOWA APPROACH" in 2012 later known as FARAPULSE Inc., which was later acquired by Boston Scientific in 2020.

Pulsed Field Ablation (PFA) is based on the premise of irreversible electroporation, where trains of high voltage, short duration energy are pulsed to create an electric field of substantial strength to injure tissue. The principle of electroporation has been used in a wide variety of practices ranging from gene therapy to tumor ablation but has only recently been applied to cardiac ablation. It is the unique properties of the cell membrane that are manipulated during electroporation. Cell membrane is composed of a phospholipid bilayer that is stabilized by Van der Waals forces that allow for aqueous pores to form in the membrane due to molecular water interactions across the cell membrane. The application of an electric field amplifies the molecular interaction of the water molecules across the cell membrane disrupting the Van der Walls forces of the phospholipid bilayer to create aqueous pores. If an electric field of substantial strength and duration is applied to the cell, these aqueous pores can become stabilized resulting in permanent disruption to the permeability of the cell membrane resulting in an apoptotic like cell death, which is termed irreversible electroporation or PFA (**Figure 4**).

RF ablation is associated with very low rate of complications but include pulmonary vein stenosis, atrio-esophageal fistula. Similarly Cryoablation is associated with low rate of complications as well but include phrenic nerve palsy. In contrast during PFA ultra rapid (microseconds to nanoseconds) electrical energy is delivered to destabilize cell membrane by forming irreversible nanoscale pores resulting in ell death, however threshold field strength for tissue necrosis is different for different tissues such as myocardium, blood vessels, nerve fibers thus rendering a great advantage of tissue selectivity. This differential tissue sensitivity to pulsed electrical fields is believed to decrease collateral damage. This single shot ablation technology in addition to being associated with clinical safety, success and durability has significantly reduced procedural time [41].

So far there have been three Multicenter studies three multicenter studies with PFA system: (IMPULSE [A Safety and Feasibility Study of the IOWA Approach Endocardial Ablation System to Treat Atrial Fibrillation], PEFCAT [A Safety

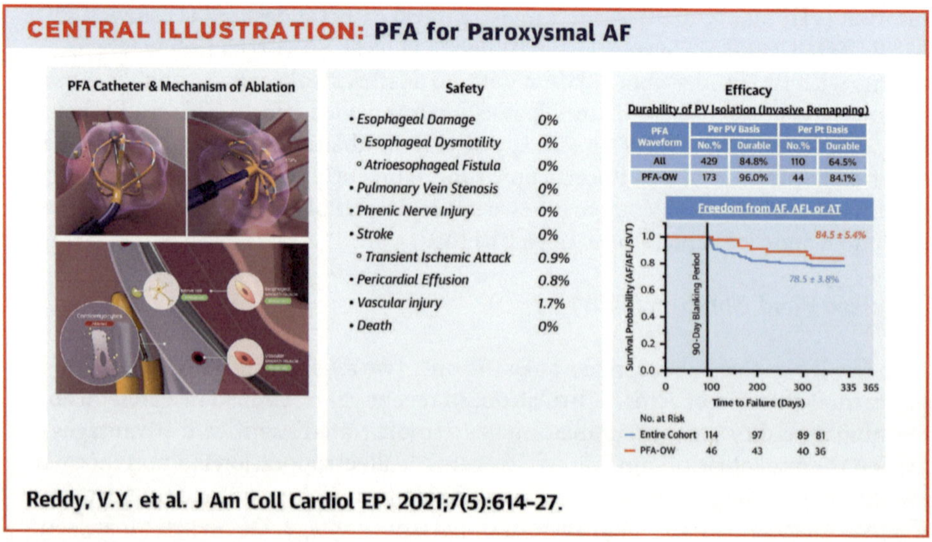

Figure 4.
Figure adopted from Reddy [41].

and Feasibility Study of the FARAPULSE Endocardial Ablation System to Treat Paroxysmal Atrial Fibrillation], and PEFCAT II [Expanded Safety and Feasibility Study of the FARAPULSE Endocardial Multi Ablation System to Treat Paroxysmal Atrial Fibrillation]). Reddy et al. [41] reported 1 year outcome of PFA in patients with PAF from these three trials. In a patient cohort of 121 patients, acute PVI with PFA was achieved in 100% of patients, primary adverse event occurred in 2.5% of patients (2 pericardial effusion, 1 transient ischemic attack, 1 hematoma), Freedom from recurrence of any atrial arrhythmia at 1 year was around 78%. In >100 patients and with 5 operators, the mean procedure times were only 96.2 ± 30.3 min, inclusive of ~20 min of voltage mapping time after PVI which is faster than procedure times with other technologies. With increased operator experience and elimination of voltage mapping, procedure times should improve further. PVI with a "single-shot" PFA catheter results in excellent PVI durability and acceptable safety with a low 1-year rate of atrial arrhythmia recurrence ushering in a new era in the front of modern day advanced Atrial Fibrillation management.

3.5 Cryoablation for atrial fibrillation

An alternative mode of PAF ablation is Cryoablation. STOP AF [42] trial compared Cryoablation and AAD and demonstrated the safety and effectiveness of Cryoablation therapy as an alternative to antiarrhythmic medication for the treatment of patients with symptomatic PAF, for whom at least one AAD has failed. RF ablation requires operator skill and training and longer time for catheter navigation to complete point by point ablation around the pulmonary veins. In contrast, cryoballoon is a balloon catheter which is positioned inside pulmonary vein and with good occlusion, with a single Cryo application pulmonary vein isolation can be achieved rather simply with short procedure time. FIRE and ICE trial [43] compared both technologies (RF vs. Cryo ablation) and found Cryoablation was non inferior to radiofrequency ablation with respect to efficacy, no significant difference in overall safety between two methods. The mean total procedure time was shorter in the cryoballoon group than in the radiofrequency group (124 vs. 141 min, $P < 0.001$), as was the left atrial dwell time (the length of time the catheter was present in the left atrium during the procedure). The mean total fluoroscopy time was shorter in the radiofrequency group than in the cryoballoon group (17 vs. 22 min, $P < 0.001$) due to navigational capabilities utilizing 3D electroanatomic mapping system with RF ablation. Though both methods (RF vs. Cryo) had similar outcomes in terms of safety, Incidence of Phrenic nerve Injury was slightly

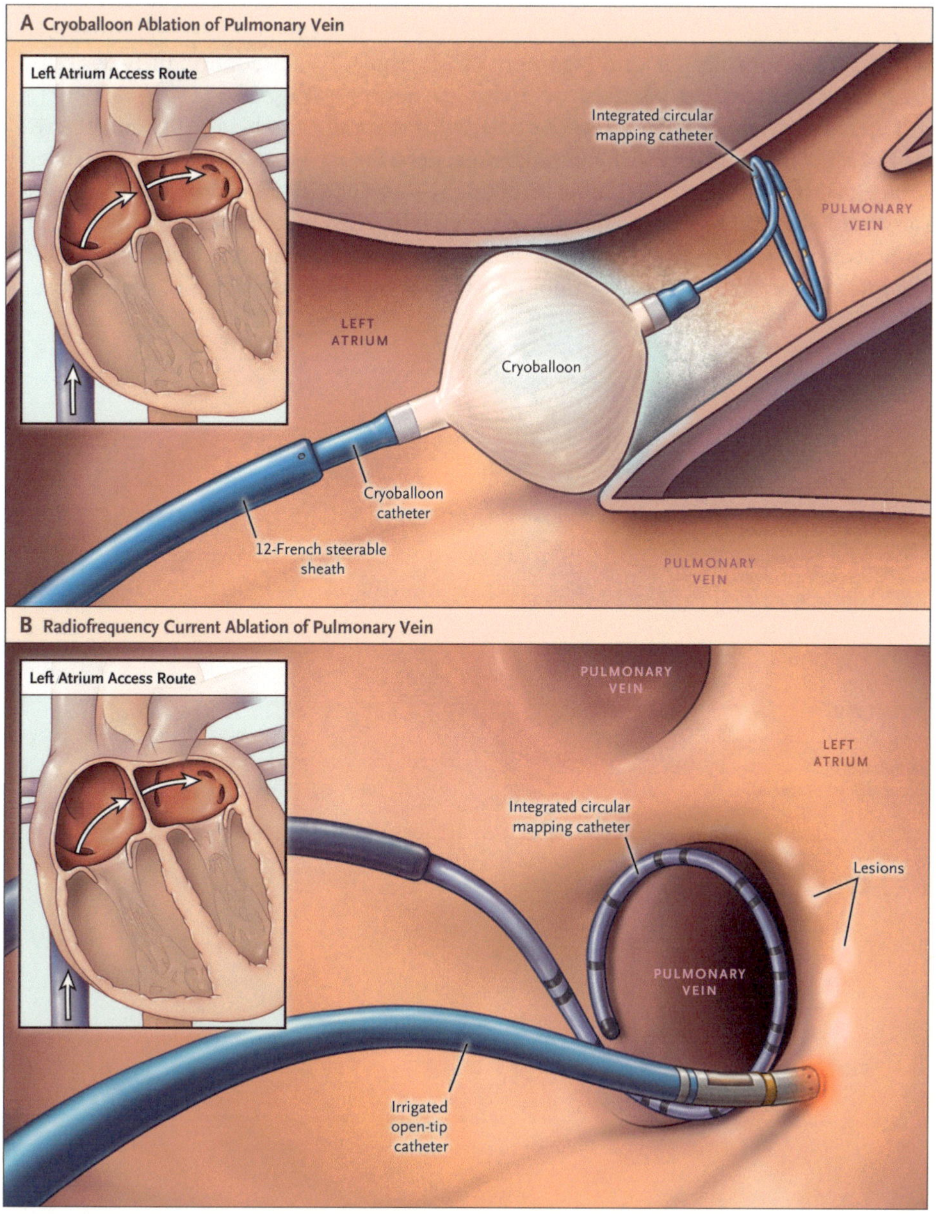

Figure 5.
Cryoballoon ablation system. There is an integrated circular mapping catheter. Balloon is inflated in the pulmonary vein and single shot application of subzero temperature is delivered to the pulmonary vein antrum. Bottom figure shows an RF ablation catheter which delivers heat energy with a point by point application around the pulmonary vein antrum. Picture courtesy FIRE AND ICE trial investigators [43].

higher in Cryoablation group, but this was substantially lower compared to reported incidence of Phrenic nerve injury in STOP AF trial group (**Figure 5**).

3.6 Cardio-neural alablation

Role of Autonomic nervous system in initiation and maintenance of AF has been a great area of interest to understand the pathophysiology of AF. Intrinsic autonomic nervous system [44] is believed to comprise of primarily 5 major ganglionated plexi (GP) located in the epicardial fat pads- superior left GP, Inferior Left GP, Anterior Right GP, Inferior right GP and Ligament of Marshal). GPs predominantly contain parasympathetic neurons but also sympathetic neurons (**Figure 6**).

It is challenging to localize GP with endocardial mapping and hence ablation effectiveness has remained controversial. One technique described to localize major GP is to elicit AV block with High frequency stimulation (HFS) [46, 47]. GPs are consistently located in areas of Left atrial fractionated atrial potential (LA FAP) [44, 46–52] commonly seen around coumadin ridge LAA-Left PV region, ligament of marshall, superior left FAP area, inferoposterior FAP, anterior right FAP. HFS at Cycle length 50 ms, 12–15 V, 10 ms

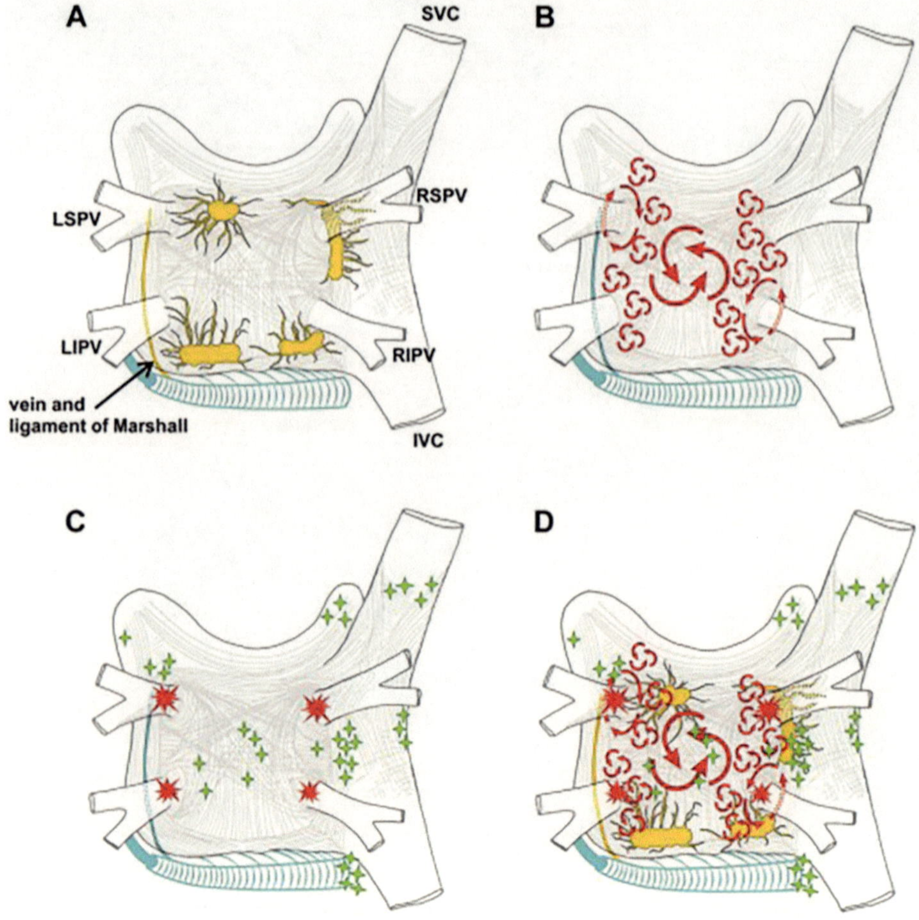

Figure 6.
Schematic diagram of major ganglionate Plexi (shown in yellow) and axons. Picture adopted from [45].

pulse width is delivered to [47, 52] and if AV block is seen (increase in R-R interval >50% during AF) and RF ablation is performed at each site exhibiting a positive HFS response. Ablation of each of the five GP areas usually requires 2–12 (median 6) RF applications. 124,582. HFS is not very sensitive to identify GP. There are other markers such as onset of PV fire from PV other than adjacent GP. There is also significant interplay between GP. AV block is mediated by inferior right GP, hence HFS of other GPs activate Inferior Right GP which innervates the AV node. If a GP is ablated along the course to Inferior Right GP, HFS may not elicited AV block. So it is usually advisable to ablate GP in the order starting with Marshal tract, superior Left, anterior right, inferior left and finally inferior right.

Pokushalov et al. showed regional ablation at the anatomic sites of the left atrial GP can be safely performed and enables maintenance of sinus rhythm in 71% of patients with paroxysmal AF for a 12-month period [53]. Katritsis et al. [54] randomized 242 patients with Paroxysmal AF into PVI alone with circumferential antral lesions, GP ablation alone, and combination of PVI with GP ablation. Freedom from AF or AT was achieved in 44 (56%), 39 (48%), and 61 (74%) patients in the PVI, GP, and PVI + GP groups, respectively ($P = 0.004$ by log-rank test). Study concluded that addition of GP ablation to PVI confers a significantly higher success rate compared with either PVI or GP alone in patients with PAF. Pokushalov et al. [55] conducted an RCT in persistent/long standing persistent AF patients including 264 patients randomized into two ars: PVI + Linear Line (LL) ($n = 132$) and PVI + GP ($n = 132$) to see whether GP or LL ablation can be a better adjunct to PVI. Sinus rhythm at 12 months (47% vs. 54%) and 3 years (34% vs. 49%) were found to be higher in the PVI + GP group. On the other hand, PVI + LL ablation group had higher incidence of Left Atrial Flutter.

Driessen et al. in AFACT [56] study compared surgical epicardial GP ablation in addition to PVI and found no improvement in outcome.

Current HRS/EHRA expert consensus states that usefulness of ablation of autonomic ganglia as an initial or repeat ablation strategy for paroxysmal, persistent, and long-standing persistent AF is not well established (Class IIb, LOE B-NR).

4. Changing landscape of safety and efficacy of catheter ablation at current era

AF ablation is a relatively complex procedure with approximately 4.5% risk of a major complication and is only available in specialized centers. But currently, this procedure is being increasingly offered to patients, and even sicker patients. With early recognition and prevention of complications, advances in technology, increased operator experience, AF ablation has become a more widely and frequently performed safe and effective procedure with low complication rates.

An updated worldwide survey on safety and efficacy of catheter ablation of AF in humans was conducted by Cappato et al. [57] between 2003 and 2006 on 20,825 procedures amongst 16,309 patients.

Complications associated with catheter ablation of Atrial Fibrillation (**Table 3**):

Vascular access complications such as hematoma, arteriovenous fistula, pseudoaneurysm etc. are low nowadays due to almost universal use of ultrasound guided vascular access. Various esophageal temperature monitoring probes (e.g. CIRCA) or Esophageal cooling devices are available that has reduced the rate of catastrophic complications like atrio-esophageal fistula.

3-D Electroanatomic mapping (EAM) and high definition (HD) mapping in the modern era has significantly improved efficacy and safety of ablation and has reduced

Type of complication	No. of patients	Rate, %
Death	25	0.15
Tamponade	213	1.31
Pneumothorax	15	0.09
Hemothorax	4	0.02
Sepsis, abscesses, or endocarditis	2	0.01
Permanent diaphragmatic paralysis	28	0.17
Total femoral pseudoaneurysm	152	0.93
Total artero-venous fistulae	88	0.54
Valve damage/requiring surgery	11/7	0.07
Atrium-esophageal fistulae	6	0.04
Stroke	37	0.23
Transient ischemic attack	115	0.71
PV stenoses requiring intervention	48	0.29
Total	741	4.54

Table 3.
Procedural risks and complication rates with catheter ablation of atrial fibrillation.

procedural time and fluoroscopy time. There are 3 mapping systems widely available CARTO (Biocense Webster Inc., Diamond Bar, California), EnSite NavX (St Jude Medical, St Paul, Minnesota), Rhythmia (Boston Scientific Inc., Marlborough, MA, USA). Pre procedural imaging, cardiac CT or MRI, integration with 3-D mapping systems further allows for increased procedural accuracy and safety. Phased array Intracardiac Echocardiogram is routinely used to aid in the visualization of cardiac anatomy, esophageal proximity to the posterior LA, pulmonary vein anatomy, catheter navigation, transeptal puncture and even tissue changes during ablation lesion delivery. The CARTO3 mapping system has the advantage of Integrated ICE (CARTOSOUND) allowing for direct integration of ICE images into the EAM system, however ICE is used in conjunction with all three mapping systems. Bidirectional steerable Navigational sheaths such as VIZIGO (Biocense Webster Inc., Diamond Bar, California) which can be visualized with EAM systems have facilitated in safe catheter navigation and reduced fluoroscopy time.

In recent years, mapping catheter technology for AF ablation has improved significantly. HD mapping catheters with unique form factors with small electrode size, spacing and orientation allows for optimized electrogram collection allowing for better assessment of electrical properties of tissue, fractionated potentials, acquire accurate anatomy/geometry, wavefront propagation etc. Deflectable mapping catheters such as PentaRay or OctaRay (CARTO, Biocense Webster), IntellaMap Orion (Boston Scientific, Marlborough, MA, USA), HD Grid (Abbott, St Pail, MN) have their unique advantages each contributing to efficacy and safety of ablation procedure. INTELLAMAP ORION High Resolution mapping catheter is a basket catheter with 64 electrodes that is capable of high definition electro-anatomical mapping providing more accurate and greater resolution. OCTARAY is a novel multielectrode catheter for high-resolution atrial mapping that has proven its utility for mapping ablation gaps and provide high resolution mapping. With improvement in software technology mapping systems are also able acquiring more points in ultrashort time, tissue proximity indicator, wavefront annotation algorithm incorporating unipolar and bipolar electrograms increasing accuracy of map and identify ablation gaps or critical targets for ablation.

With improvement in software technology, new algorithms in the mapping systems enable acquisition of data in automated, efficient, and accurate process that reduces the dependence on the system operator. Future endeavors into HD mapping of AF include the use of novel algorithms, Artifical Intelligence (AI) neural networks and non contact mapping methodologies for the identification of AF triggers and drivers.

Probably, the greatest improvement in catheter ablation has been the rapid improvement in ablation catheter and energy delivery technology. The first RF ablation catheters were non irrigated and hence were associated with risk of coagulation and char formation at the catheter tissue interface resulting in risk of embolism. With development of open irrigated ablation catheter energy delivery has become more efficient and safer. Further development in catheter technologies include the introduction of feedback mechanisms to determine catheter contact including contact force catheters and local impedance technologies. These technologies allow for assessment of catheter tissue contact, tissue proximity, electrical and mechanical coupling and quality of lesion formation.

Equipped with modern imaging, mapping or navigational ability, irrigated ablation catheters, AF catheter ablation is now emerging as a standard of care for rhythm control in modern era with shorter procedural time, reduced fluoroscopic time, low procedural complication rates probably even lesser compared to initially reported complications in the earlier publications. Current literature suggests 60–90% improvement in selected patient with medically refractory AF and 2–3 fold better than achievable with AAD [26].

5. Surgical ablation of atrial fibrillation

As mentioned above Maze III procedure has proven very effective in preventing recurrence of Atrial Fibrillation however has been limited by surgical morbidities and hence a stand alone maze procedure in the absence of any other cardiac surgery indications was difficult to justify. Since then, several other iteration of Maze III procedure has evolved most using linear lines to isolate pulmonary veins and posterior wall, though less efficacious than COX Maze procedure [58, 59]. Results from PRAGUE 12 study showed more patients stayed in sinus rhythm when surgical ablation was added to cardiac/valve surgery in patients with AF. 117 patients were randomized to receive the modified Maze surgical ablation procedure (RF or Cryo based on surgeon's preference) and 107 patients underwent surgery only. 60.2% of patients with surgical ablation were in sinus rhythm at 1 year compared to 35.5% ($P = 0.002$) and interestingly this benefit was entirely driven by improvement in long persistent and permanent AF patient group [26].

Current guideline (2017 HRS/EHRA/ECAS/APHRS/SOLAECE Expert Consensus Statement on Catheter and Surgical Ablation of Atrial Fibrillation) [45] recommendations regarding surgical ablation for AF is as follows (**Table 4**).

5.1 Hybrid convergent procedure

Although PVI has shown great efficacy in PAF, endocardial catheter ablation in patients with persistent and long standing persistent AF has reduced success rate. Posterior wall of LA is a complex anatomical structure in terms of atrial myofiber orientation which was demonstrated by Pashakhanloo et al. [60]. There is also endo-epicardial dissociation with complex 3D wavefront propagation, and endocardial mapping alone may not identify epicardial substrate, similarly endocardial ablation may not be enough to modify epicardial substrate. To overcome this limitation, a newer

COR	LOE	Recommendation
Class I	B-NR	Concomitant Open surgical ablation at the time of concomitant surgery such as Mitral Valve surgery is recommended in Symptomatic patients with Paroxysmal, Persistent or Long standing Persistent AF: 1. who are refractory or intolerant to at least one Class I or III antiarrhythmic medication 2. Prior to initiation of antiarrhythmic therapy with a Class I or III antiarrhythmic medication
Class I Class IIa	B-NR B-NR	Concomitant closed (such as CABG and AVR) surgical ablation of atrial fibrillation is recommended for symptomatic Paroxysmal, Persistent or Long standing Persistent AF 1. who are refractory or intolerant to at least one Class I or III antiarrhythmic medication 2. Prior to initiation of antiarrhythmic therapy with a Class I or III antiarrhythmic medication
Class IIa	B-NR	Stand alone and Hybrid ablation of AF is recommended for Symptomatic AF patients refractory or intolerant to at least one Class I or III antiarrhythmic medication 1. Paroxysmal: who have failed one or more attempts at catheter ablation, intolerant/refractory to AAD and prefer a surgical approach, after review of the relative safety and efficacy of catheter ablation vs. a stand-alone surgical approach. 2. Persistent and long standing persistent: who have failed one or more attempts at catheter ablation, and prefer a surgical approach, after review of the relative safety and efficacy of catheter ablation vs. a stand-alone surgical approach.

Table 4.
2017 HRS/EHRA/ECAS/APHRS/SOLAECE expert consensus on surgical ablation for AF.

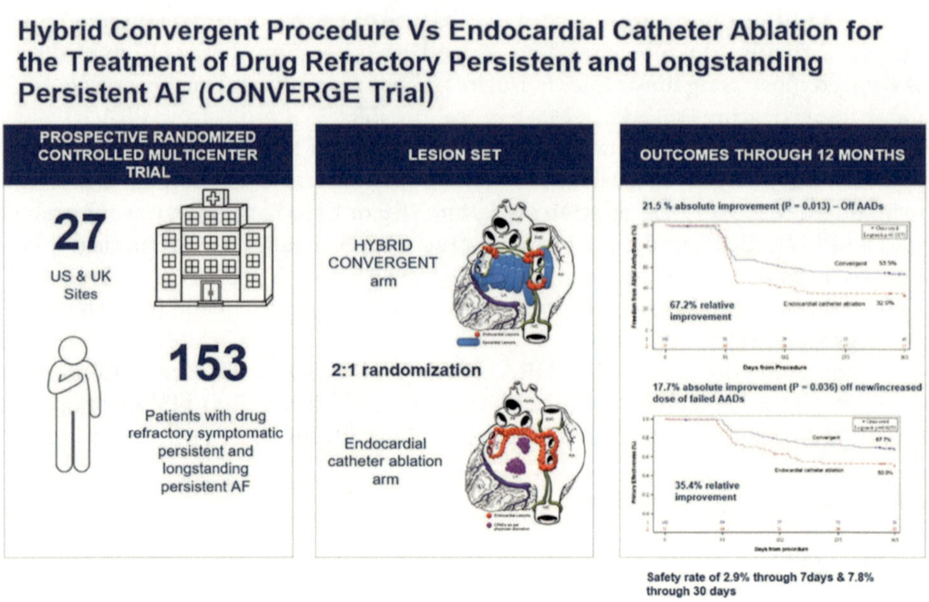

Figure 7.
Figure adopted from DeLurgio et al. [61].

hybrid convergent approach with endo-epicardial ablation was compared to endocardial ablation alone in the CONVERGENT [61] trial by DeLurgio et al. (**Figure 7**).

One-hundred fifty-three patients were randomized 2:1 to Hybrid Convergent vs. catheter ablation. Epicardial ablation was performed with unipolar radiofrequency device (EPi-Sense, AtriCure, OH). Pericardial access was gained through a transdiaphragmatic or subxiphoid approach, and the radiofrequency device was positioned inside a pericardioscopic cannula with an endoscope. Primary outcome was freedom from AF/AFl/AT without AAD or previously failed AAD without increase in dosage. Study concluded that Hybrid Convergent procedure has superior effectiveness compared to the catheter ablation for the treatment of persistent and long-standing persistent atrial fibrillation.

Both findings from PRAGUE 12 study and CONVERGENT trial provides unique insight into understanding the mechanism of Persistent and long standing persistent AF and offers new treatment options for this variety of AF which is more difficult to tackle with endocardial ablation alone.

6. Device detected atrial fibrillation

Device detected or subclinical atrial fibrillation (SCAF) is a term that broadly encompasses AT detected by cardiac implantable electronic devices (CIEDs), which include implantable cardiac monitors, dual-chamber pacemakers, dual-chamber implantable cardioverter-defibrillators, and cardiac resynchronization therapy devices. There is no consensus about role of anticoagulation in this unique group of patients, though it is believed to affect as many as one-third of the U.S. population. Current guidelines recommend OAC for stroke and systemic embolism prophylaxis in patients with non valvular atrial fibrillation based on CHADSVasc2 score irrespective of Paroxysmal, persistent/long standing persistent or permanent category. False detection may occur due to oversensing of far field R wave, noise, or runs of Premature atrial complexes (PAC) or undersensing may misdiagnose true AT and hence all device detected Atrial high response events (AHRE) require further verification by physician.

The temporal relationship between atrial fibrillation and stroke is not as well understood, and in some patients, episodes of AF are not detected until months after a stroke. Though studies like CRYSTAL AF [62] and EMBRACE [63] has shown increased trend of anticoagulation prescription by physicians amongst patients with cryptogenic stroke who has AF detected with an implantable loop monitor or an event monitor for 30 days, there was reduced trend towards starting anticoagulation amongst patients with CIED detected AF without cryptogenic stroke [64]. Multiple studies, including MOST, TRENDS, and ASSERT trials have added insight into this unique clinical situation of SCAF. Subgroup analysis of 316 patients from MOST (MOde Selection) trial in patients with sinus node dysfunction showed AHRE (atrial rate > 220 beats/min for 10 consecutive beats) was an independent predictor of mortality or nonfatal stroke and AF, indicating that pacemaker patients with sinus node dysfunction and AHRE were more than 2.5 times as likely to die or have a stroke, and were 6 times as likely to develop AF than those without AHRE [65]. TRENDS [66] study prospectively looked at 2486 patients with pacemakers or defibrillators that monitor AT/AF burden (defined as the longest total AT/AF duration on any given day during the prior 30-day period) and concluded that AT>5.5 h was significantly associated with increased risk of thromboembolic event in patients with ≥1 stroke risk factor (heart failure, hypertension, age ≥65 years, diabetes, or prior thromboembolic event) and emphasized the notion that Thromboembolism risk is a quantitative function of AT/AF burden. In the ASSERT study, subclinical episodes of AT, defined as atrial rates ≥190 beats/min lasting >6 min, were associated with an increased risk of ischemic stroke [67]. Stroke risk was incremental with longer duration of AT but similar risk between AT of 6–24 h duration, or >24 h duration, stroke risk increased with the number of subclinical AT episodes [68]. IMPACT [69] trial had a predefined anticoagulation plan. Anticoagulation protocol was initiated if AT (defined as ≥200 beats/min for 36 of 48 beats) was detected≥48 h in patients with $CHADS_2$ score ≤2 with discontinuation of anticoagulation if there were no AT recurrences detected for 30 days, CHADS2 scores of ≥3 to 4 would initiate anticoagulation for device-detected AT ≥24 h in 2 days, with discontinuation if there were no AT recurrences detected for 90 days, patients with CHADS2 scores ≥5 to 6, or with a history of prior thromboembolism were prescribed anticoagulant therapy for any AT, without discontinuation, regardless of AT recurrence [68]. Data Monitoring Committee recommended trial termination on the basis of failure to demonstrate a meaningful difference in outcome with the interventional strategy. There was no significant difference between groups in the primary outcome, which was the composite of ischemic stroke, systemic embolic, and major hemorrhagic events, or in all-cause mortality.

Guidelines are unclear about role of anticoagulation in device detected SCAF. One school hypothesizes there is lack of scientific evidence to prove benefit of anticoagulation in SCAF and there is no clear consensus regarding "how much is too much device detected AF" based on varying duration of AF seen in various trials. Other school argues that there is lack of temporal relationship between AF and stroke/thromboembolism reflecting AF is marker for increased risk of stroke or systemic thromboembolism and hence anticoagulation if initiated with detection of AF may prevent stroke. It is accepted that risk of stroke is independent of duration (Paroxysmal or persistent) of AF or symptoms of AF in patients with clinical AF and mostly governed by risk factors for stroke (e.g. CHADSVasc2 risk calculator tool). There is no answer to whether AF-related stroke risk varies on the method of AF detection e.g., 12 lead ECG, Holter monitor, Implantable loop monitor or pacemaker-defibrillator. It is established that SCAF is a common clinical situation and eventually on longitudinal follow up many of these patients eventually develop clinical AF. Thus device detected AF offers an opportunity for closer monitoring of this patient population, and initiation of anticoagulation should be based on risk of stroke guided by tools as $CHADSVsac_2$ score profile after patient-physician discussion based on patient preference and values.

7. Non pharmacological stroke prevention/left atrial appendage occlusion

AF increases the risk of stroke [70] 5 times, irrespective of Paroxysmal, Persistent or permanent nature, symptomatic or asymptomatic status, and thromboembolism occurring with AF is associated with a greater risk of recurrent stroke, more severe disability, and mortality. Role of anticoagulation in prevention of stroke and systemic embolism have been already established (**Figure 8**).

New target specific oral anticoagulation agents such as Dabigatran, Rivaroxaban, Apixaban, Edoxaban and Betrixaban are available. Some have shown superior efficacy over Coumadin while others proved non inferior to coumadin. Reversal agents

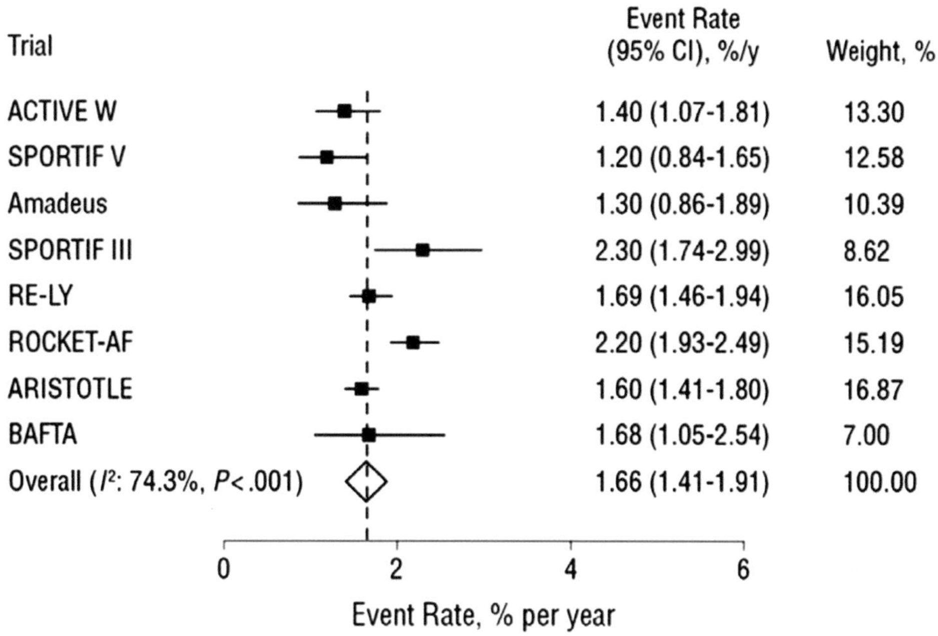

Figure 8.
Meta-analysis of landmark trials showing role of anticoagulation in patients with non valvular atrial fibrillation.

are available. However, bleeding risk is a major concern with use of anticoagulation. Coumadin has narrow time in therapeutic range, multiple drug and food interaction and need for lifelong anticoagulation. People who cannot tolerate oral anticoagulation but are at increased risk of stroke requires non pharmacological stroke prevention. LAA is the primary source of thromboembolism in AF [71] and obliteration of LAA is associated with reduction of stroke. There are two different approaches available for LAA occlusion percutaneously. One is plugging the appendage with a device like WATCHMAN (Boston Scientific, Natick, MA) or Amplatzer cardiac plug (St. Jude Medical, Plymouth, MN). Other approach is to ligate the LAA with an epicardial approach using LARIAT device, (SentreHEART, Redwood City, CA) which requires transeptal and subxiphoid approach. With LARIAT device, Acute closure rate is high with low rate of leak however procedure success is limited due to bleeding.

Holmes et al. [72, 73] published the initial safety and feasibility data in 66 patients who underwent LAA occlusion with WATCHMAN. No strokes occurred during follow up despite discontinuation of anticoagulation, there were two patients with device embolization, two cardiac tamponade, one air embolism, two deaths not related to device. But in subsequent larger RCT and LAAO registries complication rates were much lower with increasing operator experience. PROTECT AF [72, 73] was a large multi center RCT that compared LAAO with WATCHMAN device to anticoagulation with coumadin. After 3.8 years of follow up, LAAO showed non inferiority and also superiority compared to coumadin in preventing combined outcome of stroke and embolism, cardiovascular death, all cause death. Similarly, PREVAIL [74] trial assessed the safety and efficacy of LAAO in patients with Non valvular Atrial Fibrillation (NVAF) compared to long term warfarin therapy and showed LAAO was noninferior to warfarin for ischemic stroke prevention or SE >7 days' post-procedure, and procedural safety has significantly improved. There are two large registries now CAP (Continued access to PROTECT-AF) and CAP 2 (continued access to PREVAIL) that provides long term safety and efficacy of LAAO with WATCHMAN for stroke prevention. Data from these two longest and largest registries showed LAAO with WATCHMAN device is safe and effective therapy for stroke prevention in NVAF. Though PROTECT-AF data showed non inferiority and superiority of LAAO over Warfarin, complication rates were higher. This was addressed in the subsequent PREVAIL trial. There was however, unexpectedly low rate of ischemic stroke in Warfarin cohort. This was believed to be due to relatively small patient population followed for relatively short duration. A subsequent metanalysis of these two trials by Reddy et al. [75] showed ischemic stroke/Systemic embolism rate was numerically higher with LAA Closure, but this difference did not reach statistical significance (HR: 1.71; $P = 0.080$). However, differences in hemorrhagic stroke, disabling/fatal stroke, cardiovascular/unexplained death, all-cause death, and post-procedure bleeding favored LAA closure. Procedure safety has significantly improved after next generation of WATCHMAN device called WATCHMAN FLX was designed. PINNACLE FLX [76] study enrolled around 400 patients who underwent WATCHMAN FLX implantation. Primary efficacy endpoint was effective LAA closure defined by ≤5 mm peridevice flow, secondary efficacy endpoint was ischemic stroke or systemic embolism at 24 months, primary safety end point was all cause death, ischemic stroke/systemic embolism, device or procedure related adverse event requiring surgery or major end-vascular intervention within 7 days following the procedure or hospital discharge whichever is later. Ischemic stroke occurred in 0.5%, no death, pericardial effusion or device embolization were reported, implant success rate was 99%. 96.2% of patients were able to discontinue NOAC at 45 day follow up. The next generation device WATCHMAN FLX has shown further safety and efficacy of the procedure overcoming the initial limitations of LAAO seen during PROTECT-AF trial. Currently there is another ongoing large RCT which has completed enrolling patients (OPTIONS clinical trial) that will compare safety and effectiveness of LAA closure to OAC therapy after AF ablation. CHAMPION-AF trial is ongoing and comparing WATCHMAN FLX as a first line stroke risk reduction therapy vs. NOAC for NVAF patients.

Surgical ligation of LAA is usually performed with internal sewing or stapling. Procedure is limited by bleeding, and residual stump which acts a source of thrombus. AtriClip is an external clip that is a newer technique for surgical LAA occlusion under direct visualization in patients undergoing open Cardiothoracic surgical procedure. 3.5 year follow up showed stable clips, no LAA thrombi, or neurological event, and no neck >1 cm.

Current AHA/ACC/HRS guidelines recommend as follows for non pharmacological stroke prevention (**Table 5**).

COR	LOE	Rcommendation
Class IIb	B-NR	Percutaneous LAA occlusion may be considered in patients with AF at increased risk of stroke who have contraindications to long-term anticoagulation
Class IIb	B-NR	Surgical occlusion of the LAA may be considered in patients with AF undergoing cardiac surgery, as a component of an overall heart team approach to the management of AF.

Table 5.
AHA/ACC/HRS recommendation for non pharmacological stroke prevention.

8. Conclusion

Atrial Fibrillation is a commonly prevalent arrhythmia with increasing prevalence and incidence. There have been significant development in the field of AF treatment in recent years which has changed physician's outlook towards this growing arrhythmia epidemic. With several recent RCTs and other wealth of scientific evidence, benefits of early rhythm control is being increasingly recognized. Catheter ablation is safe and effective, feasible in controlling AF burden, improving quality of life, reduce hospitalization, improve heart failure symptoms and exercise capacity, reduce hospitalization and offers mortality benefit in patients with reduced LV systolic function. Mapping and ablation technology has significantly improved in recent years and is still growing and evolving. Various modalities for ablation such as RF along with its different strategic ramifications such as VoM alcohol ablation, substrate modification, Cryo-Ablation, PFA or Hybrid Convergent procedures have opened up more treatment choices available to both Paroxysmal and Persistent/Long standing persistent Atrial Fibrillation patients. Stroke prevention with LAA occlusion has proven effective and successful in patients who cannot tolerate or have a contraindication for long term anticoagulation.

Abbreviations/acronyms

ACC	American College of Cardiology
AF	Atrial Fibrillation
AFl	Atrial Flutter
AHA	American Heart Association
AHRE	Atrial High response event
AT	Atrial tachycardia
AAD	Antiarrhythmic drug
CFAE	Complex Fractionated Atrial Electrogram
CIED	Cardiac Implantable Electronic Device
CTI	Cavo tricuspid Isthmus
CHF	Congestive Heart Failure
COR	Category of Recommendation
EAM	Electroanatomic mapping
EF	Ejection Fraction
HD	High Definition
HF	Heart Failure
HFS	High Frequency Stimulation
HFrEF	Heart Failure with Reduced Ejection Fraction
HFpEF	Heart Failure with Preserved Ejection Fraction
HPSD	High Power Short Duration
HRS	Heart Rhythm Society
ITT	Intention to Treat
LA	Left Atrium
LAA	Left Atrial Appendage
LAAO	Left Atrial Appendage Occlusion
LA FAP	Left Atrial Fractionated atrial potential
LL	Linear Line
LOE	Level of Evidence

LPLD	Low Power Long Duration
LVEF	Left Ventricular Ejection Fraction
NOAC	Novel oral anticoagulant
NVAF	Non valvular Atrial Fibrillation
PAC	Premature Atrial Complex
PAF	Paroxysmal Atrial Fibrillation
PFA	Pulsed Field Ablation
PV	Pulmonary vein
PVI	Pulmonary Vein Isolation
RA	Right Atrium
RCT	Randomized Clinical Trial
RF	Radiofrequency
SCAF	Subclinical Atrial Fibrillation
SVC	Superior Vena Cava
vHPSD	Very High Power Short Duration
VoM	Vein of Marshall
W	Watts

Author details

Nayanjyoti Kaushik[1*], James Arter Chapman[2], Andrew Gillaspie[2], Stephen Ackerman[1], Peter Gallagher[1], Deobrat Mallick[3] and Steven J. Bailin[4]

1 CHI Health Nebraska Heart Institute, Lincoln, NE, USA

2 Boston Scientific, Inc., Marlborough, MA, USA

3 Christus Spohn Hospital, Corpus Christi, TX, USA

4 University of Iowa Hospitals, Iowa City, IA, USA

*Address all correspondence to: kaushik_nayan@yahoo.co.in

References

[1] Packer DL, Mark DB, Robb RA, et al. Effects of Catheter Ablation vs Antiarrhythmic Drug Therapy on Mortality, Stroke, Bleeding, and Cardiac arrest among patients with Atrial Fibrillation. The CABANA Randomized clinical trial. Journal of the American Medical Association. 2019;**321**(13):1261-1274. DOI: 10.1001/jama.2019.0693

[2] Ott A, Breteler MM, de Bruyne MC et al. Atrial Fibrillation and dementia in a population based study. The Rotterdam Study. 1997;**28**(2):316-321. DOI: 10.1161/01.str.28.2.316. PMID: 9040682

[3] Benjamin EJ, Wolf PA, D'Agostino RB, et al. Impact of Atrial Fibrilation on the risk of death: the Framingham Heart Study. Circulation. 1998;**98**(10):946-952. DOI: 10.1161/01.cir.98.10.946. PMID: 9737513

[4] January CT, Calkins H, Stevenson WG, et al. 2014 AHA/ACC/HRS Guideline for the Management of Patients With Atrial Fibrillation: A Report of the American College of Cardiology/American Heart Association Task Force on Practice Guidelines and the Heart Rhythm Society. DOI: 10.1016/j.jacc.2014.03.022

[5] Olshansky B, Rosenfeld LE, Warner AL, et al. Journal of the American College of Cardiology. 2004;**43**(7):1201-1208. DOI: 10.1016/j.jacc.2003.11.032 PMID: 15063430

[6] Van Gelder IC, Hagens VE, et al. The New England Journal of Medicine. 2002;**347**:1834-1840. DOI: 10.1056/NEJMoa021375

[7] Singh BN, Singh SN, Domenic JR, et al. The New England Journal of Medicine. 2005;**352**:1861-1872. DOI: 10.1056/NEJMoa041705

[8] Hagens VE, Ranchor AV, Van Sonderen E, et al. Journal of the American College of Cardiology. 2004;**43**(2):241-247

[9] Bunch TJ, Crandall BG, Weiss JP, et al. Journal of Cardiovascular Electrophysiology. 2011;**22**(8):839-845. DOI: 10.1111/j.1540-8167.2011.02035.x Epub 2011 Mar 15. PMID: 21410581

[10] Cosio FG, Aliot E, Botto GL, et al. Europace. 2008;**10**(1):21-27. DOI: 10.1093/europace/eum276 Epub December 17, 2007. PMID: 18086696

[11] Kirchhof P, Bax J, Blomstrom-Lundquist C, Calkins H, et al. Early and comprehensive management of atrial fibrillation: Executive summary of the proceedings from the 2nd AFNET-EHRA consensus conference 'research perspectives in AF'. European Heart Journal. 2009;**30**(24):2969-277c. DOI: 10.1093/eurheartj/ehp235. PMID: 19535417

[12] Van Gelder IC, Haegeli LM, Brandes A, et al. Europace. 2011;**13**(11):1517-1525. DOI: 10.1093/europace/eur192 Epub July 22, 2011. PMID: 21784740; PMCID: PMC3198586

[13] Cosedis Nielsen J, Johannessen A, Raatikainen P, et al. The New England Journal of Medicine. 2012;**367**(17):1587-1595. DOI: 10.1056/NEJMoa1113566 PMID: 23094720

[14] Morillo CA, Verma A, Connolly SJ, et al. Journal of the American Medical Association. 2014;**311**(7):692-700. DOI: 10.1001/jama.2014.467 Erratum in: Journal of the American Medical Association. 2014;**311**(22):2337. Erratum in: Journal of the American Medical Association. 2021;**326**(4):360. PMID: 24549549

[15] Roy D, Talajic M, Nattel S, Wyse DG, et al. The New England Journal of Medicine. 2008;**358**(25):2667-2677. DOI: 10.1056/NEJMoa0708789 PMID: 18565859

[16] Khan MN, Jaïs P, Cummings J, Di Biase L, Natale A, et al. The New England Journal of Medicine. 2008;**359**(17):1778-1785. DOI: 10.1056/NEJMoa0708234 PMID: 18946063

[17] MacDonald MR, Connelly DT, Hawkins NM, et al. Radiofrequency ablation for persistent atrial fibrillation in patients with advanced heart failure and severe left ventricular systolic dysfunction: A randomised controlled trial. Heart. 2011;**97**(9):740-747. DOI: 10.1136/hrt.2010.207340 Epub November 4, 2010. PMID: 21051458

[18] Jones DG, Haldar SK, Hussain W, et al. Journal of the American College of Cardiology. 2013;**61**(18):1894-1903. DOI: 10.1016/j.jacc.2013.01.069 Epub March 7, 2013. PMID: 23500267

[19] Chen MS, Marrouche NF, Khaykin Y, et al. Journal of the American College of Cardiology. 2004;**43**(6):1004-1009. DOI: 10.1016/j.jacc.2003.09.056 PMID: 15028358

[20] Di Biase L, Santangeli P, Lakkireddy D, Jais P, Haissaguerre M, Natale A, et al. Circulation. 2016;**133**(17):1637-1644. DOI: 10.1161/CIRCULATIONAHA.115.019406 Epub March 30, 2016. PMID: 27029350

[21] Marrouche NF, Brachmann J, Andresen D, et al. Catheter ablation for atrial fibrillation with heart failure. The New England Journal of Medicine. 2018;**378**(5):417-427. DOI: 10.1056/NEJMoa1707855 PMID: 29385358

[22] Kirchhof P, Camm AJ, Goette A, et al. The New England Journal of Medicine. 2020;**383**(14):1305-1316. DOI: 10.1056/NEJMoa2019422 Epub August 29, 2020. PMID: 32865375

[23] Wazni OM, Dandamudi G, Sood N, et al. The New England Journal of Medicine. 2021;**384**(4):316-324. DOI: 10.1056/NEJMoa2029554 Epub November 16, 2020. PMID: 33197158

[24] 2019 AHA/ACC/HRS Focused Update of the 2014 AHA/ACC/HRS Guideline for the Management of Patients With Atrial Fibrillation: A Report of the American College of Cardiology/American Heart Association Task Force on Clinical Practice Guidelines and the Heart Rhythm Society

[25] Cox JL, Schuessler RB, D'Agostino HJ Jr, et al. The surgical treatment of atrial fibrillation. III. Development of a definitive surgical procedure. The Journal of Thoracic and Cardiovascular Surgery. 1991;**101**(4):569-583 PMID: 2008095

[26] Issa ZF, Miller JM, Zipes DP. Clinical Arrhythmology and Electrophysiology: A Companion to Braunwald's Heart Disease. 2nd ed; Elsevier

[27] Haïssaguerre M, Jaïs P, Shah DC, et al. The New England Journal of Medicine. 1998;**339**(10):659-666. DOI: 10.1056/NEJM199809033391003 PMID: 9725923

[28] Pappone C, Rosanio S, Oreto G, et al. Circumferential radiofrequency ablation of pulmonary vein ostia: A new anatomic approach for curing atrial fibrillation. Circulation. 2000;**102**:2619-2628 11085966

[29] Bisbal F, Alarcón F, Ferrero-De-Loma-Osorio A, et al. Journal of Cardiovascular Electrophysiology. 2019;**30**(9):1483-1490. DOI: 10.1111/jce.14000 Epub June 6, 2019. PMID: 31115940

[30] Bunch TJ, May HT, Bair TL, et al. Heart Rhythm. 2013;**10**(9):1257-1262. DOI: 10.1016/j.hrthm.2013.05.013 Epub May 20, 2013. PMID: 23702238

[31] Hussein AA, Saliba WI, Barakat A, et al. Circulation: Arrhythmia and Electrophysiology. 2016;**9**(1):e003669. DOI: 10.1161/CIRCEP.115.003669 PMID: 26763227; PMCID: PMC5349298

[32] Verma A, Jiang CY, Betts TR, et al. Approaches to catheter ablation for persistent atrial fibrillation. The New England Journal of Medicine. 2015;**372**(19):1812-1822. DOI: 10.1056/NEJMoa1408288 PMID: 25946280

[33] Clarnette JA, Brooks AG, Sanders P, et al. Europace. 2018;**20**(FI_3):f366-f376. DOI: 10.1093/europace/eux297 PMID: 29267853

[34] Di Biase L, Burkhardt JD, Al-Ahmad A, Lakkireddy D, Natale A, et al. Left atrial appendage isolation in patients with longstanding persistent AF undergoing catheter ablation: BELIEF trial. Journal of the American College of Cardiology. 2016;**68**(18):1929-1940. DOI: 10.1016/j.jacc.2016.07.770 PMID: 27788847

[35] Valderrábano M, Peterson LE, Swarup V, et al. Journal of the American Medical Association. 2020;**324**(16):1620-1628. DOI: 10.1001/jama.2020.16195 PMID: 33107945; PMCID: PMC7592031

[36] Bhaskaran A, Chik W, Pouliopoulos J, et al. Europace. 2017;**19**(5):874-880. DOI: 10.1093/europace/euw077 PMID: 27207815

[37] Kotadia ID, Williams SE, O'Neill M. High-power, short-duration radiofrequency ablation for the treatment of AF. Arrhythmia & Electrophysiology Review. 2020;**8**(4):265-272. DOI: 10.15420/aer.2019.09 PMID: 32685157; PMCID: PMC7358956

[38] Winkle RA, Jais P, Natale A, et al. Low complication rates using high power (45-50 W) for short duration for atrial fibrillation ablations. Heart Rhythm. 2019;**16**(2):165-169. DOI: 10.1016/j.hrthm.2018.11.031 PMID: 30712645

[39] Reddy VY, Grimaldi M, Natale A, et al. JACC: Clinical Electrophysiology. 2019;**5**(7):778-786. DOI: 10.1016/j.jacep.2019.04.009 Epub May 8, 2019. PMID: 31320006

[40] HIgh Power Short Duration Radiofrequency Ablation or Cryoballoon Ablation for Paroxysmal Atrial Fibrillation (HIPAF). ClinicalTrials.gov Identifier: NCT04855890

[41] Reddy VY, Dukkipati SR, Neuzil JP, et al. Pulsed field ablation of paroxysmal atrial fibrillation: 1-Year outcomes of IMPULSE, PEFCAT, and PEFCAT II. JACC: Clinical Electrophysiology. 2021;**7**(5):614-627. DOI: 10.1016/j.jacep.2021.02.014 Epub April 28, 2021. PMID: 33933412

[42] Packer DL, Kowal RC, Wheelan KR, et al. Journal of the American College of Cardiology. 2013;**61**(16):1713-1723. DOI: 10.1016/j.jacc.2012.11.064 Epub March 21, 2013. PMID: 23500312

[43] Kuck KH, Brugada J, Fürnkranz A, et al. The New England Journal of Medicine. 2016;**374**(23):2235-2245. DOI: 10.1056/NEJMoa1602014 Epub April 4, 2016. PMID: 27042964

[44] Kawashima T. The autonomic nervous system of the human heart with special reference to its origin, course, and peripheral distribution. Anatomy and Embryology (Berlin). 2005;**209**(6):425-438. DOI: 10.1007/s00429-005-0462-1 Epub May 11, 2005. PMID: 15887046

[45] 2017 HRS/EHRA/ECAS/APHRS/SOLAECE Expert Consensus Statement on Catheter and Surgical Ablation of Atrial Fibrillation

[46] Hou Y, Scherlag BJ, Lin J, et al. Ganglionated plexi modulate extrinsic cardiac autonomic nerve input: Effects on sinus rate, atrioventricular conduction, refractoriness, and inducibility of atrial fibrillation. Journal of the American College of Cardiology. 2007;**50**(1):61-68. DOI: 10.1016/j.jacc.2007.02.066 Epub June 18, 2007. PMID: 17601547

[47] Nakagawa H, Scherlag BJ, Patterson E, et al. Pathophysiologic basis of autonomic ganglionated plexus ablation in patients with atrial fibrillation. Heart Rhythm. 2009;**6**(12 Suppl):S26-S34. DOI: 10.1016/j.hrthm.2009.07.029 Epub October 24, 2009. PMID: 19959140

[48] Po SS, Nakagawa H, Jackman WM. Localization of left atrial ganglionated plexi in patients with atrial fibrillation. Journal of Cardiovascular Electrophysiology. 2009;**20**(10):1186-1189. DOI: 10.1111/j.1540-8167.2009.01515.x Epub June 26, 2009. PMID: 19563367

[49] Patterson E, Po SS, Scherlag BJ, Lazzara R. Triggered firing in pulmonary veins initiated by in vitro autonomic nerve stimulation. Heart Rhythm. 2005;**2**(6):624-631. DOI: 10.1016/j.hrthm.2005.02.012 PMID: 15922271

[50] Scherlag BJ, Nakagawa H, Jackman WM, et al. Electrical stimulation to identify neural elements on the heart: Their role in atrial fibrillation. Journal of Interventional Cardiac Electrophysiology. 2005;**13**(Suppl. 1):37-42. DOI: 10.1007/s10840-005-2492-2 PMID: 16133854

[51] Patterson E, Lazzara R, Szabo B, et al. Sodium-calcium exchange initiated by the Ca^{2+} transient: An arrhythmia trigger within pulmonary veins. Journal of the American College of Cardiology. 2006;**47**(6):1196-1206. DOI: 10.1016/j.jacc.2005.12.023 Epub February 23, 2006. PMID: 16545652

[52] Stavrakis S, Nakagawa H, Po SS, et al. The role of the autonomic ganglia in atrial fibrillation. JACC: Clinical Electrophysiology. 2015;**1**(1-2):1-13. DOI: 10.1016/j.jacep.2015.01.005 PMID: 26301262; PMCID: PMC4540352

[53] Pokushalov E, Romanov A, Artyomenko S, et al. Left atrial ablation at the anatomic areas of ganglionated plexi for paroxysmal atrial fibrillation. Pacing and Clinical Electrophysiology. 2010;**33**(10):1231-1238. DOI: 10.1111/j.1540-8159.2010.02800.x PMID: 20546147

[54] Katritsis DG, Pokushalov E, Romanov A, et al. Autonomic denervation added to pulmonary vein isolation for paroxysmal atrial fibrillation: A randomized clinical trial. Journal of the American College of Cardiology. 2013;**62**(24):2318-2325. DOI: 10.1016/j.jacc.2013.06.053 Epub August 21, 2013. PMID: 23973694

[55] Pokushalov E, Romanov A, Katritsis DG, et al. Ganglionated plexus ablation vs linear ablation in patients undergoing pulmonary vein isolation for persistent/long-standing persistent atrial fibrillation: A randomized comparison. Heart Rhythm. 2013;**10**(9):1280-1286. DOI: 10.1016/j.hrthm.2013.04.016 Epub April 19, 2013. PMID: 23608592

[56] Driessen AHG, Berger WR, Krul SPJ, et al. Ganglion plexus ablation in advanced atrial fibrillation: The AFACT study. Journal of the American College of Cardiology. 2016;**68**(11):1155-1165. DOI: 10.1016/j.jacc.2016.06.036 PMID: 27609676

[57] Cappato R, Calkins H, Chen SA, et al. Circulation: Arrhythmia and Electrophysiology. 2010;**3**(1):32-38. DOI: 10.1161/CIRCEP.109.859116 Epub December 7, 2009. PMID: 19995881

[58] Shen J, Bailey MS, Damiano RJ Jr. The surgical treatment of atrial fibrillation. Heart Rhythm. 2009;**6**(8 Suppl):S45-S50. DOI: 10.1016/j.hrthm.2009.05.019 Epub May 22, 2009. PMID: 19631907; PMCID: PMC2760330

[59] Mack MJ. Current results of minimally invasive surgical ablation for isolated atrial fibrillation. Heart Rhythm. 2009;**6**(12 Suppl):S46-S49. DOI: 10.1016/j.hrthm.2009.08.020 PMID: 19959143

[60] Pashakhanloo F, Herzka DA, Ashikaga H, et al. Myofiber architecture of the human atria as revealed by submillimeter diffusion tensor imaging. Circulation: Arrhythmia and Electrophysiology. 2016;**9**(4):e004133. DOI: 10.1161/CIRCEP.116.004133 PMID: 27071829; PMCID: PMC7035884

[61] DB DL, Crossen KJ, Calkins H. Results of the CONVERGE clinical trial. Circulation: Arrhythmia and Elecrophysiology. 2020;**13**:e009288

[62] Sanna T, Diener HC, Passman RS, et al. Cryptogenic stroke and underlying atrial fibrillation. The New England Journal of Medicine. 2014;**370**(26):2478-2486. DOI: 10.1056/NEJMoa1313600 PMID: 24963567

[63] Gladstone DJ, Spring M, Dorian P, et al. Atrial fibrillation in patients with cryptogenic stroke. The New England Journal of Medicine. 2014;**370**(26):2467-2477. DOI: 10.1056/NEJMoa1311376 PMID: 24963566

[64] Healey JS, Martin JL, Connolly SJ, et al. The Canadian Journal of Cardiology. 2013;**29**(2):224-228. DOI: 10.1016/j.cjca.2012.08.019 Epub November 9, 2012. PMID: 23142343

[65] Glotzer TV, Hellkamp AS, Zimmerman J, et al. Circulation. 2003;**107**(12):1614-1619. DOI: 10.1161/01.CIR.0000057981.70380.45 Epub March 24, 2003. PMID: 12668495

[66] Glotzer TV, Daoud EG, Wyse DG, et al. The relationship between daily atrial tachyarrhythmia burden from implantable device diagnostics and stroke risk: The TRENDS study. Circulation: Arrhythmia and Electrophysiology. 2009;**2**(5):474-480. DOI: 10.1161/CIRCEP.109.849638 Epub August 4, 2009. PMID: 19843914

[67] Healey JS, Connolly SJ, Gold MR, et al. The New England Journal of Medicine. 2012;**366**(2):120-129. DOI: 10.1056/NEJMoa1105575 Erratum in: The New England Journal of Medicine. March 10, 2016;**374**(10):998. PMID: 22236222

[68] Chen-Scarabelli C, Scarabelli TM, Ellenbogen KA, et al. Journal of the American College of Cardiology. 2015;**65**(3):281-294. DOI: 10.1016/j.jacc.2014.10.045 PMID: 25614426

[69] Healey JS, Lopes RD, Connolly SJ, et al. European Heart Journal. 2015;**36**(26):1640-1642. DOI: 10.1093/eurheartj/ehv159 Epub May 2, 2015. PMID: 25935876

[70] Wolf PA, Abbott RD, Kannel WB. Atrial fibrillation as an independent risk factor for stroke: The Framingham study. Stroke. 1991;**22**(8):983-988. DOI: 10.1161/01.str.22.8.983 PMID: 1866765

[71] Blackshear JL, Odell JA. Appendage obliteration to reduce stroke in cardiac

surgical patients with atrial fibrillation. The Annals of Thoracic Surgery. 1996;**61**(2):755-759. DOI: 10.1016/0003-4975(95)00887-X PMID: 8572814

[72] Sick PB, Schuler G, Hauptmann KE, Holmes DR, et al. Initial worldwide experience with the WATCHMAN left atrial appendage system for stroke prevention in atrial fibrillation. Journal of the American College of Cardiology. 2007;**49**(13):1490-1495. DOI: 10.1016/j.jacc.2007.02.035 Epub March 21, 2007. PMID: 17397680

[73] Reddy VY, Sievert H, Halperin J, Doshi SK, Holmes DR, et al. Journal of the American Medical Association. 2014;**312**(19):1988-1998. DOI: 10.1001/jama.2014.15192. Erratum in: Journal of the American Medical Association. March 10, 2015;**313**(10):1061. PMID: 25399274

[74] Holmes DR Jr, Kar S, Reddy VY, et al. Prospective randomized evaluation of the watchman left atrial appendage closure device in patients with atrial fibrillation versus long-term warfarin therapy: The PREVAIL trial. Journal of the American College of Cardiology. 2014;**64**(1):1-12. DOI: 10.1016/j.jacc.2014.04.029 Erratum in: Journal of the American College of Cardiology September 16, 2014;**64**(11):1186. PMID: 24998121

[75] Reddy VY, Doshi SK, Kar S, et al. 5-year outcomes after left atrial appendage closure: From the PREVAIL and PROTECT AF trials. Journal of the American College of Cardiology. 2017;**70**(24):2964-2975. DOI: 10.1016/j.jacc.2017.10.021 Epub November 4, 2017. PMID: 29103847

[76] Kar S, Doshi SK, Sadhu A, Reddy VY, et al. Circulation. 2021;**143**(18):1754-1762. DOI: 10.1161/CIRCULATIONAHA.120.050117 Epub April 6, 2021. PMID: 33820423

Chapter 7

Atrial Fibrillation in Heart Failure: Rate or Rhythm Control Strategy

Anggia Chairuddin Lubis, Dian Andina Munawar and Muhammad Munawar

Abstract

Atrial fibrillation and heart failure are intimately related as they shared the same risk factors, unsurprisingly they commonly coexist and complicate each other. Management of atrial fibrillation in heart failure is usually simplified into rate or rhythm control strategy, as each offers its advantages and limitations. Pharmacological rate and rhythm control strategy has been compared for the last decades; however, as more nonpharmacological approach raised as viable option has driven the management strategy discussion even further. On the other hand, heart failure understanding is also evolving and more detailed classification has been made based on left ventricular function. Justification for rate or rhythm control strategy should be individualized predicated on clinical phenotype. Moreover, the chosen strategy should be flexible and can be adjusted if the preferred strategy is ineffective.

Keywords: atrial fibrillation, heart failure, rate control, rhythm control, pharmacological strategy, catether ablation

1. Introduction

Atrial fibrillation (AF) and heart failure (HF) commonly coexist that frequently complicate one another and exert a significant detrimental effect on cardiovascular health and well-being [1]. Altered left ventricular (LV) functions may be the substrate for most HF spectrum, heart failure with reduced ejection fraction (HFrEF) and heart failure with preserved ejection fraction (HFpEF), but in some instances, HFpEF may be the consequence of a failing left atrium (LA) including AF. It is believed that AF can induced and worsened HF due to: (1) elevated resting heart rate and exaggerated response during exercise result in reduction of diastolic filling time, leading to cardiac output reduction. Irregularity of the ventricular response will affect the cardiac output even further [2]. (2) Heart rate irregularity with calcium mishandling, even in AF with the absence of tachycardia we can observe potential deleterious interaction of AF and LV function; (3) loss of atrial contraction associated with sympathetic activation contributing to limited ventricular filling and increased filling pressures, functional mitral regurgitation, and diastolic function [3, 4]. Studies in AF patients have shown the atria structural remodeling changes; however, the impact of arrhythmia chronicity and the structural remodeling is not well understood; adaptive (dedifferentiation of cardiomyocytes) and maladaptive (degeneration of cells with replacement fibrosis) features are the changes mainly concern [5].

Management strategy of rate or rhythm control strategy has been thoroughly discussed over the last decades. Rate control strategy is considered as first-line therapy in most AF; however, the evidence keeps evolving. The decision to treat AF with a rate versus rhythm control strategy depends on multiple factors, including: medical comorbidities, age, and lifetime exposure to the risks and side effects of treatments; the duration and type of AF; and concomitant medications. Based on recent clinical trials, treatment strategies for patients with AF are increasingly focused on rhythm control by catheter ablation compared with rate control therapy [1, 3]. This chapter will discuss each strategy further.

2. Role of rate control strategy

AF is frequently considered a primary cause of arrhythmia-induced cardiomyopathy. AF by itself in the absence of tachycardia causes impaired excitation-contraction coupling associated with increased levels of reactive oxygen species and CaMKII-dependent depression of systolic Ca^{2+} release, clinically frequently observed as impaired ventricular function [3]. Furthermore, limited evidence suggests that controlled ventricular rate during AF does not predict the reversibility of cardiomyopathy. This has raised the question whether well-controlled heart rate in AF can reverse this process. However, early studies failed to demonstrate rhythm control superiority over rate control strategy [4, 6].

Traditionally rate control strategy is the primary option in AF with or without HF [7, 8]. AFFIRM is the landmark trial to exposed rhythm control strategy and offers no survival benefit over rate control strategy while more adverse drug effects were also seen. These findings were later confirmed by other studies [6, 9]. Nevertheless, extrapolation from these studies to patients with HF should be done with caution.

In patients with HF, similar results were also observed in landmark AF trials. AF-CHF (rhythm control vs. rate control for atrial fibrillation and heart failure) trial was the first randomized study to examine the effect of rate versus rhythm control strategy in a heart failure population; it showed pharmacological rhythm control is not superior to rate control for the prevention of cardiac death and hospitalization for heart failure, therefore extends the findings of AF without HF. Of note, most of these trials were performed before the era of catheter ablation for AF. The need for effective therapy to maintain sinus rhythm while minimizing toxicity is the highlight of the difficulty with currently available antiarrhythmic drug (AAD) [2, 4, 10, 11]. Nevertheless, up-to-date rate control strategy remained as first option in AF with HF.

2.1 Drug selection for rate control strategy

There are several atrioventricular nodal blockers that can be used to obtain rate control; beta-blockers, non-dyhidropyridine calcium channel blockers, cardiac glycosides, and (in rare circumstances) low-dose amiodarone. Pharmacological rate control strategies are different for patients with HFrEF and HFpEF.

Beta-blockers and digoxin can be used in those with HFrEF. Beta-blockers are well known as of the HFrEF management pillars, suited well in HF with AF comorbidity.

Beta-blockers may both control the ventricular rate to AF and improve survival of HFrEF. A meta-analysis showed that the effect of beta-blockers on outcome in HF patients with reduced left ventricular ejection fraction (LVEF) who have AF is less than in those who have sinus rhythm. This result does not suggest that there is no benefit of beta-blockers in HF and AF, but rather highlights the benefits of sinus rhythm in patients with HF [8, 12, 13]. Digoxin slows ventricular response to AF through enhancement of vagal tone and therefore is less effective in states of increased sympathetic tone such as exercise or worsening heart failure. However, digoxin may be used as adjunct therapy to beta-blockers as it exerts a synergistic effect with beta-blockers after single therapeutic option failed to achieve optimal target heart rate. Of note, digoxin should be used with caution because of its potential deleterious effects [2, 7, 14, 15].

The non-dihydropyridine calcium-channel blockers include diltiazem and verapamil, beta-blockers, and digoxin are all viable options in HFpEF. The non-dihydropyridine calcium-channel blockers are effective rate control agents; however, because of their negative inotropic effect, they may be not tolerated at optimal dose required for optimal ventricular rate control and increased mortality in HFrEF. Beta-blockers were more successful than calcium-channel blockers in achieving rate control (70% vs. 54%, consecutively) when used alone or in combination with digitalis. Amiodarone is also another option for rate control in both forms of HF, but limited only to acute settings [1, 8, 16].

2.2 Optimal AF target heart rate in HF

Optimal target heart rate in AF is informed by several factors, including symptom management, optimization of functional capacity, and preventing HF exacerbation and tachycardia-induced cardiomyopathy. High ventricular rates are clearly harmful and can result in symptoms and especially in patients with preexisting HF [17]. The decision to use of strict or lenient as optimal level of heart rate control in AF and HF is essential in management strategy.

A major concern with lenient heart rate control is the decompensation episode of HF may occur; however, this concern was not confirmed [18]. Strict rate control cannot be advocated over lenient rate control for patients with preserved LV function; however, it potentially offers clinical benefit in patients with AF and HFrEF, but this remains unproven. The latest European Society of Cardiology (ESC) guidelines recommend a lenient rate control of <100–110 bpm as initial approach; however, tight rate control strategy can be considered in case with persistent symptoms or cardiac dysfunction likely related to tachycardia. It should be noted that these criteria were not based on strong clinical evidence [7, 8].

2.3 Pace and ablate strategy

Atrioventricular node ablation with permanent pacemaker placement remains an important option, it should be undertaken with caution. One concern of pharmacological rate and rhythm control strategies is the risk of pauses or symptomatic bradycardia during AF or at the time of AF conversion to sinus (conversion pauses). Another common scenario is patient coexists with sinus node dysfunction, a permanent pacemaker is usually required during significant bradycardia [1, 19].

Effective rate control is often hard to achieve in patients with or without pacemaker in situ. In patients without pacemaker, symptomatic pauses during AF or at the time of conversion of paroxysmal AF to sinus rhythm make effective rate control not possible. Ineffectiveness of rate controlling drugs or intolerance to the drugs at doses that result in adequate rate control is indication for the use of permanent pacemaker. In these strategies, combination of AV nodal radiofrequency ablation and permanent pacemaker implantation can be performed as definitive strategy with a high success rate [19, 20].

In patients with symptomatic AF and rapid ventricular response refractory to pharmacological therapy, radiofrequency atrioventricular nodal ablation with subsequent pacemaker placement can improve cardiac performance. In the subgroup of patients with heart failure, the degree of improvement for LVEF and NYHA class was even greater [21]. However, long-term outcomes of the "pace and ablate" strategy have been less favorable [22]. AV nodal ablation typically results in nearly 100% right ventricular (RV) pacing, which can induce ventricular dyssynchrony and worsen systolic function. A large body of evidence has emerged recently that underscores the harmful effects of long-term right ventricular pacing.

A study showed that patients who underwent AV nodal ablation with cardiac resynchronization (CRT) achieved significantly better symptomatic relief with improvement in their LV function [23]. The CRT impact on new onset AF is controversial. CRT can reverse the remodeling of the ventricle, improve the regurgitation of the mitral valve, and theoretically reduce the incidence of new-onset AF [2]. Recently, multiple studies showed conduction system pacing (His bundle pacing and left bundle branch area pacing) is not inferior to CRT. However, the current evidence of conduction system pacing is still limited and neither has been evaluated as robustly as CRT [24–26]. AV nodal ablation in the presence of let bundle branch area pacing lead is associated with a higher success rate and fewer acute and chronic lead related complications compared with His bundle pacing [27].

AV nodal ablation and pacing for patients with AF have not been found to worsen survival in comparison with drug therapy for AF [28]. Unfortunately, this pace and ablate strategy results in permanent pacemaker dependence and irreversible. It should be performed only as a last resort when other rate and/or rhythm control strategies have been failed or are contraindicated.

3. Role of rhythm control strategy

Previous trials cast skepticism over the hard end point benefit of sinus-rhythm maintenance in patients with and without heart failure. Trials including patients with HF and comparing rate control and rhythm control strategies with the pharmacological approach failed to show mortality benefit of one strategy over the other [10, 29]. Consequently, previous guidelines have limited recommendations for catheter ablation (CA) in patients with HF: when tachycardiomyopathy is suspected, with pharmacological rate control the accepted standard treatment [30].

CA for AF has emerged as alternative strategy to pharmacological rhythm control, as it significantly reduces the risk of death, stroke, and hospitalization compared with medical therapy alone [13, 31, 32]. It is a well-established option for symptomatic AF that is resistant to drug therapy in patients with otherwise normal cardiac function [8].

EAST-AFNET 4 (Early Treatment of Atrial Fibrillation for Stroke Prevention Trial) has emphasized that aggressive rhythm control (with either CA or drugs) early in the course of AF reduced adverse cardiovascular outcomes compared with usual care. The effects of an early rhythm-control strategy on the primary outcome appeared to be generally consistent across predefined subgroups, including patients with or without HF [33].

In the field of CA in HF, various studies have shown that ablation is associated with positive outcomes in patients with HF. Important to note is that initial series were often single-center studies that included a limited number of patients with limited follow-up, and its effectiveness in improving rates of hard primary end points such as death or the progression of HF was not tested [34, 35]. More recently, larger trials with substantial longer duration of follow-up and cardiovascular endpoints as well as sinus rhythm maintenance have been conducted.

3.1 Medical vs catheter ablation for rhythm control

AF-CHF and DIAMOND-CHF trials found no difference in mortality between AAD therapy and rate control. The mortality benefit of AADs in previous trials may have been limited by their adverse effects [10, 29]. AADs may not be as efficacious as catheter ablation in providing freedom from AF in patients with HF, and there is increasing evidence that the maintenance of sinus rhythm is the key determinant of survival [11].

Several trials have reported improvements in soft end points with catheter ablation. The AATAC and CAMTAF trials showed that CA was superior to medical treatment in maintaining sinus rhythm and improving LVEF. The trial also showed a favorable effect on rates of death and hospitalization for HF [36, 37].

CASTLE-AF is notable because previous trials comparing CA versus standard medical therapy predominantly reported improvement in soft endpoints (symptoms, QOL, or surrogate endpoints). In the CASTLE-AF trial, ablation for AF in HF was superior to medical therapy in reducing composite death and hospitalization. The benefit of all-cause mortality in the ablation group was driven by lower rate of cardiovascular mortality. The mortality benefit of ablation did not emerge until after 3 years. Pursuing rhythm control with catheter ablation proved to be of significant benefit with regard to outcomes [38].

However, CASTLE-AF enrolled a highly selected population, 363 of 3013 patients were not blinded, had crossovers between the two treatment strategies, and the number of events observed was low. Both CASTLE-AF and CABANA showed a highly significant effect of catheter ablation on patients' symptoms [38–40].

CASTLE-AF trial's results are likely driven by two factors: Firstly, CA procedural risks have fewer risks and long-term toxicities than medical therapy. Secondly, ablation is more effective in reducing AF burden. One of the proposed mechanisms behind the improvement in prognosis in the patients treated with CA is that it significantly reduced total AF burden. Post-hoc analysis showed that AF burden below 50% after 6 months of CA was associated with an improved outcome. Another potential explanation is that part of the patients had a tachycardiomyopathy. Longer periods of sinus rhythm may, therefore, be a mechanism to improve outcome eventually [11, 38].

Furthermore, the absence of ventricular LGE on cardiac MRI imaging was associated with a greater improvement in LVEF and a higher likelihood of normalization of left ventricular function. These findings indicate that in these patients, AF may either significantly contribute to, or indeed be entirely responsible for, ventricular dysfunction [13]. Meta-analyses showed that AF ablation was associated with average

LVEF improvement ranged between 11% and 13% illustrating the advantage of AF ablation. Improvement in LVEF was most pronounced in patients with non-ischemic cardiomyopathy [41–43].

Another interesting observation was seen in AF and HFpEF. Both conditions shared similar risk factors, including hypertension, sleep apnea, advanced age diastolic dysfunction, and obesity. The prevalence of HFpEF in AF ranges from 8% to 24%, and AF was found in ~20–30% patients with HFpEF [40]. Restoration and maintenance of sinus rhythm in patients with comorbid AF and HFpEF improve hemodynamic parameters, BNP, and symptoms associated with HFpEF [44].

4. Potential deleterious effects of pharmacological therapy

Understanding and identification of drug deleterious effects are also another important issue for management consideration. Digoxin's ability to reduce heart rate and improving LV function is very tempting; however, digoxin's potential deleterious effects such as arrhythmogenic potential, narrow therapeutic window, increased sympathetic activity, and risk for serious drug interaction. A meta-analysis of nonrandomized trials showed digoxin used in HF and AF is associated with an increased risk of all-cause mortality [15]. Moreover, the use of pharmacological rhythm control also brings risk. Amiodarone carries the risk of thyroid, pulmonary, and hepatic toxicity. Dofetilide therapy is also known for prolonging QT interval and higher rate of torsade de pointes [45, 46].

5. Catheter ablation vs pace and ablate

Biventricular pacing was found to be superior to right ventricular pacing after atrioventricular-node ablation [47]. However, PABA-CHF trial has shown that CA for AF provides superior morphological and functional improvements compared with atrioventricular-node ablation with biventricular pacing in patients with HF who had drug-refractory AF [20].

6. Catheter ablation strategy

The improvement in LVEF observed following CA may largely be dependent on successful rhythm restoration, rather than the mode of restoration, which enables regular ventricular filling time and coordinated atrial contraction [46]. CA by pulmonary vein isolation (PVI) is proven as the best technique for AF ablation, as no proven benefit shown by additional ablation.

After Haissaguerre et al. found that radiofrequency ablation on PV is efficient in treating AF in 1998, no additional ablation technique (posterior wall ablation, linear lines or ablation of complex fractional aytrial electrograms) has been proven consistently to improve ablation efficacy; however, additional ablation can be done up to the operator's discretion. Future research endeavors should be performed into the field of high-power short duration, pulsed field ablation, and hybrid/convergent AF ablation strategies in patients with AF and HF [11, 48].

7. Catheter ablation patient selection

In selecting patients with HF for catheter ablation of AF, the increased risk of major peri-procedural events must be carefully weighed against the potential improvement in systolic function, quality of life, and functional status.

AF ablation can be performed safely and long-term prognosis can improve, especially in patients with a tachycardiomyopathy, that is, without other demonstrable underlying heart disease. Based on the post-hoc analysis of CASTLE-AF, patients with NYHA I/II and non-ischemic etiology of HF appear to benefit the most, suggesting that early intervention might be beneficial [49].

Furthermore, enlargement of the atria and evidence of fibrosis on CMR are an indication of poor candidate for CA. A trial of cardioversion with electrical cardioversion and/or amiodarone can be used if there is a doubt whether patients may benefit from sinus rhythm [11].

8. Catheter ablation for AF limitation

There are small but nonzero procedural risks that must be taken into account when considering CA, including risks of stroke (0.5–1%) and tamponade (1–2%); however, a second ablation is frequently required [1]. CA for AF and HF was performed at centers with experienced ablationists in most landmark trials, and the results thus may not be reproducible in all centers [20].

9. Conclusion

In the management of AF in HFrEF, there is insufficient evidence in favor of a strategy of rhythm control with antiarrhythmic drugs vs. rate control in patients with HF and AF. Pharmacological rate control strategy remained as leading option in AF and HF. More evidence is needed to weigh the short-term risks of catheter ablation versus the long-term risks associated with antiarrhythmic therapy in those with AF and HFrEF. Notably, this has led to recent guideline changes suggesting that CA may be considered as first-line therapy in patients with AF and HFrEF (Class I recommendation). Pace and ablate option should be keep as last resort, because this becomes pacemaker-dependent and irreversible. Conduction system pacing as alternative pacing site in AF and HF should be an interesting area to watch in the future. On the other hand, pharmacological approach remained as preferred strategy in HFpEF; non-dihydropyridine calcium-channel blockers are the additional alternative medication compared with HFrEF. Evidence on nonpharmacological approach for AF in HFpEF is still limited.

Author details

Anggia Chairuddin Lubis[1], Dian Andina Munawar[2,3] and Muhammad Munawar[2,3]*

1 Faculty of Medicine, Universitas Sumatera Utara, Sumatera Utara, Indonesia

2 Faculty of Medicine, Department of Cardiology and Vascular Medicine, Universitas Indonesia, Jakarta, Indonesia

3 Binawaluya Cardiac Centre, Jakarta, Indonesia

*Address all correspondence to: muna286@gmail.com

References

[1] Carlisle MA, Fudim M, DeVore AD, Piccini JP. Heart failure and atrial fibrillation, like fire and fury. JACC Heart Failure. 2019;7(6):447-456. DOI: 10.1016/j.jchf.2019.03.005

[2] Anter E, Jessup M, Callans DJ. Atrial fibrillation and heart failure: Treatment considerations for a dual epidemic. Circulation. 2009;**119**(18):2516-2525. DOI: 10.1161/CIRCULATIONAHA.108.821306

[3] Pabel S, Knierim M, Stehle T, et al. Effects of atrial fibrillation on the human ventricle. Circulation Research. 2022;**130**(7):994-1010. DOI: 10.1161/CIRCRESAHA.121.319718

[4] Huizar JF, Ellenbogen KA, Tan AY, Kaszala K. Arrhythmia-induced cardiomyopathy: JACC state-of-the-art review. Journal of American Colege ofl Cardiology. 2019;**73**(18):2328-2344. DOI: 10.1016/j.jacc.2019.02.045

[5] Thijssen VL, Ausma J, Liu GS, Allessie MA, van Eys GJ, Borgers M. Structural changes of atrial myocardium during chronic atrial fibrillation. Cardiovascular Pathology. 2000;**9**(1): 17-28. DOI: 10.1016/s1054-8807(99) 00038-1

[6] de Denus S, Sanoski CA, Carlsson J, Opolski G, Spinler SA. Rate vs rhythm control in patients with atrial fibrillation: A meta-analysis. Archives in Internal Medicine. 2005;**165**(3):258-262. DOI: 10.1001/archinte.165.3.258

[7] McDonagh TA, Metra M, Adamo M, et al. 2021 ESC Guidelines for the diagnosis and treatment of acute and chronic heart failure. European Heart Journal. 2021;**42**(36):3599-3726. DOI: 10.1093/eurheartj/ehab368

[8] Hindricks G, Potpara T, Dagres N, et al. 2020 ESC Guidelines for the diagnosis and management of atrial fibrillation developed in collaboration with the European Association for Cardio-Thoracic Surgery (EACTS): The Task Force for the diagnosis and management of atrial fibrillation of the European Society of Cardiology (ESC) Developed with the special contribution of the European Heart Rhythm Association (EHRA) of the ESC. European Heart Journal. 2021;**42**(5):373-498. DOI: 10.1093/eurheartj/ehaa612

[9] Wyse DG, Waldo AL, DiMarco JP, et al. A comparison of rate control and rhythm control in patients with atrial fibrillation. New England Journal of Medicine. 2002;**347**(23):1825-1833. DOI: 10.1056/NEJMoa021328

[10] Roy D, Talajic M, Nattel S, et al. Rhythm control versus rate control for atrial fibrillation and heart failure. New England Journal of Medicine. 2008;**358**(25):2667-2677. DOI: 10.1056/NEJMoa0708789

[11] Mulder BA, Rienstra M, Van Gelder IC, Blaauw Y. Update on management of atrial fibrillation in heart failure: A focus on ablation. Heart. 2022;**108**(6):422-428. DOI: 10.1136/heartjnl-2020-318081

[12] Rienstra M, Damman K, Mulder BA, Van Gelder IC, McMurray JJ, Van Veldhuisen DJ. Beta-blockers and outcome in heart failure and atrial fibrillation: A meta-analysis. JACC Heart Failure. 2013;**1**(1):21-28. DOI: 10.1016/j.jchf.2012.09.002

[13] Prabhu S, Taylor AJ, Costello BT, et al. Catheter ablation versus medical rate control in atrial fibrillation and

systolic dysfunction: The CAMERA-MRI Study. Journal of American College of Cardiology. 2017;**70**(16):1949-1961

[14] Farshi R, Kistner D, Sarma JS, Longmate JA, Singh BN. Ventricular rate control in chronic atrial fibrillation during daily activity and programmed exercise: A crossover open-label study of five drug regimens. Journal of the American College of Cardiology. 1999;**33**(2):304-310. DOI: 10.1016/s0735-1097(98)00561-0

[15] Bavishi C, Khan AR, Ather S. Digoxin in patients with atrial fibrillation and heart failure: A meta-analysis. International Journal of Cardiology. 2015;**188**:99-101. DOI: 10.1016/j.ijcard.2015.04.031

[16] Olshansky B, Rosenfeld LE, Warner AL, et al. The Atrial Fibrillation Follow-up Investigation of Rhythm Management (AFFIRM) study: Approaches to control rate in atrial fibrillation. Journal of the American College of Cardiology. 2004;**43**(7):1201-1208. DOI: 10.1016/j.jacc.2003.11.032

[17] Bohm M, Swedberg K, Komajda M, et al. Heart rate as a risk factor in chronic heart failure (SHIFT): The association between heart rate and outcomes in a randomised placebo-controlled trial. Lancet. 2010;**376**(9744):886-894

[18] Van Gelder IC, Groenveld HF, Crijns HJ, et al. Lenient versus strict rate control in patients with atrial fibrillation. New England Journal of Medicine. 2010;**362**(15):1363-1373. DOI: 10.1056/NEJMoa1001337

[19] Heist EK, Mansour M, Ruskin JN. Rate control in atrial fibrillation: Targets, methods, resynchronization considerations. Circulation. 2011;**124**(24):2746-2755. DOI: 10.1161/CIRCULATIONAHA.111.019919

[20] Khan MN, Jais P, Cummings J, et al. Pulmonary-vein isolation for atrial fibrillation in patients with heart failure. New England Journal of Medicine. 2008;**359**(17):1778-1785. DOI: 10.1056/NEJMoa0708234

[21] Manolis AG, Katsivas AG, Lazaris EE, Vassilopoulos CV, Louvros NE. Ventricular performance and quality of life in patients who underwent radiofrequency AV junction ablation and permanent pacemaker implantation due to medically refractory atrial tachyarrhythmias. Journal of Interventional Cardiac Electrophysiology. 1998;**2**(1):71-76. DOI: 10.1023/a:1009721008761

[22] Hsieh MH, Tai CT, Lee SH, et al. Catheter ablation of atrial fibrillation versus atrioventricular junction ablation plus pacing therapy for elderly patients with medically refractory paroxysmal atrial fibrillation. Journal of Cardiovascular Electrophysiology. 2005;**16**(5):457-461. DOI: 10.1111/j.1540-8167.2005.40632.x

[23] Gasparini M, Auricchio A, Regoli F, et al. Four-year efficacy of cardiac resynchronization therapy on exercise tolerance and disease progression: The importance of performing atrioventricular junction ablation in patients with atrial fibrillation. Journal of American College of Cardiology. 2006;**48**(4):734-743

[24] Hua J, Wang C, Kong Q, et al. Comparative effects of left bundle branch area pacing, His bundle pacing, biventricular pacing in patients requiring cardiac resynchronization therapy: A network meta-analysis. Clinical Cardiology. 2022;**45**(2):214-223. DOI: 10.1002/clc.23784

[25] Qi J, Jia X, Wang Z. His bundle pacing for cardiac resynchronization therapy: A systematic literature

review and meta-analysis. Journal of Interventional Cardiac Electrophysiology. 2020;**59**(2):463-470. DOI: 10.1007/s10840-020-00827-6

[26] Qian Z, Zou F, Wang Y, et al. Permanent His bundle pacing in heart failure patients: A systematic review and meta-analysis. Pacing and Clinical Electrophysiology PACE. 2019;**42**(2): 139-145. DOI: 10.1111/pace.13565

[27] Pillai A, Kolominsky J, Koneru JN, et al. Atrioventricular junction ablation in patients with the conduction system pacing leads: A comparison of his bundle vs left bundle branch area pacing leads. Heart Rhythm. 26 Mar 2022;**19**(7):1116-1123. DOI: 10.1016/j.hrthm.2022.03.1222

[28] Ozcan C, Jahangir A, Friedman PA, et al. Long-term survival after ablation of the atrioventricular node and implantation of a permanent pacemaker in patients with atrial fibrillation. New England Journal of Medicine. 2001;**344**(14):1043-1051. DOI: 10.1056/NEJM200104053441403

[29] Torp-Pedersen C, Moller M, Bloch-Thomsen PE, et al. Dofetilide in patients with congestive heart failure and left ventricular dysfunction. Danish Investigations of Arrhythmia and Mortality on Dofetilide Study Group. New England Journal of Medicine. 1999;**341**(12):857

[30] Kirchhof P, Benussi S, Kotecha D, et al. 2016 ESC Guidelines for the management of atrial fibrillation developed in collaboration with EACTS. Europace. 2016;**18**(11):1609-1678. DOI: 10.1093/europace/euw295

[31] Saglietto A, De Ponti R, Di Biase L, et al. Impact of atrial fibrillation catheter ablation on mortality, stroke, and heart failure hospitalizations: A meta-analysis. Journal of Cardiovascular Electrophysiology. 2020;**31**(5):1040-1047. DOI: 10.1111/jce.14429

[32] Morillo CA, Verma A, Connolly SJ, et al. Radiofrequency ablation vs antiarrhythmic drugs as first-line treatment of paroxysmal atrial fibrillation (RAAFT-2): A randomized trial. JAMA. 2014;**311**(7):692-700. DOI: 10.1001/jama.2014.467

[33] Kirchhof P, Camm AJ, Goette A, et al. Early rhythm-control therapy in patients with atrial fibrillation. New England Journal of Medicin. 2020;**383**(14):1305-1316. DOI: 10.1056/NEJMoa2019422

[34] Jones DG, Haldar SK, Hussain W, et al. A randomized trial to assess catheter ablation versus rate control in the management of persistent atrial fibrillation in heart failure. Journal of American College of Cardiology. 2013;**61**(18):1894-1903. DOI: 10.1016/j.jacc.2013.01.069

[35] MacDonald MR, Connelly DT, Hawkins NM, et al. Radiofrequency ablation for persistent atrial fibrillation in patients with advanced heart failure and severe left ventricular systolic dysfunction: A randomised controlled trial. Heart. 2011;**97**(9):740-747. DOI: 10.1136/hrt.2010.207340

[36] Di Biase L, Mohanty P, Mohanty S, et al. Ablation versus amiodarone for treatment of persistent atrial fibrillation in patients with congestive heart failure and an implanted device: Results from the AATAC multicenter randomized trial. Circulation. 2016;**133**(17):1637-1644

[37] Hunter RJ, Berriman TJ, Diab I, et al. A randomized controlled trial of catheter ablation versus medical treatment of atrial fibrillation in heart failure (the CAMTAF trial). Circulation. Arrhythmia and Electrophysiology. 2014;**7**(1):31-38. DOI: 10.1161/CIRCEP.113.000806

[38] Marrouche NF, Kheirkhahan M, Brachmann J. Catheter ablation for atrial fibrillation with heart failure. New England Journal of Medicine. 2018;**379**(5):492

[39] Packer DL, Piccini JP, Monahan KH, et al. Ablation versus drug therapy for atrial fibrillation in heart failure: Results from the CABANA Trial. Circulation. 2021;**143**(14):1377-1390. DOI: 10.1161/CIRCULATIONAHA.120.050991

[40] Rosenfeld LE, Enriquez AD. The Cabana Trial and heart failure: Some sun and some shade. Circulation. 2021;**143**(14):1391-1393. DOI: 10.1161/CIRCULATIONAHA.120.053160

[41] Anselmino M, Matta M, D'Ascenzo F, et al. Catheter ablation of atrial fibrillation in patients with left ventricular systolic dysfunction: A systematic review and meta-analysis. Circulation. Arrhythmia and Electrophysiology. 2014;**7**(6):1011-1018. DOI: 10.1161/CIRCEP.114.001938

[42] Asad ZUA, Yousif A, Khan MS, Al-Khatib SM, Stavrakis S. Catheter ablation versus medical therapy for atrial fibrillation: A systematic review and meta-analysis of randomized controlled trials. Circulation. Arrhythmia and Electrophysiology. 2019;**12**(9):e007414. DOI: 10.1161/CIRCEP.119.007414

[43] Kheiri B, Osman M, Abdalla A, et al. Catheter ablation of atrial fibrillation with heart failure: An updated meta-analysis of randomized trials. International Journal of Cardiology. 2018;**269**:170-173. DOI: 10.1016/j.ijcard.2018.07.024

[44] Sugumar H, Nanayakkara S, Vizi D, et al. A prospective STudy using invAsive haemodynamic measurements foLLowing catheter ablation for AF and early HFpEF: STALL AF-HFpEF. European Journal of Heart Failure. 2021;**23**(5):785-796. DOI: 10.1002/ejhf.2122

[45] Trulock KM, Narayan SM, Piccini JP. Rhythm control in heart failure patients with atrial fibrillation: Contemporary challenges including the role of ablation. Journal of American College of Cardiology. 2014;**64**(7):710-721

[46] Virk SA, Bennett RG, Chow C, et al. Catheter ablation versus medical therapy for atrial fibrillation in patients with heart failure: A meta-analysis of randomised controlled trials. Heart, Lung & Circulation. 2019;**28**(5):707-718. DOI: 10.1016/j.hlc.2018.10.022

[47] Doshi RN, Daoud EG, Fellows C, et al. Left ventricular-based cardiac stimulation post AV nodal ablation evaluation (the PAVE study). Journal of Cardiovascular Electrophysiology. 2005;**16**(11):1160-1165. DOI: 10.1111/j.1540-8167.2005.50062.x

[48] Haissaguerre M, Jais P, Shah DC, et al. Spontaneous initiation of atrial fibrillation by ectopic beats originating in the pulmonary veins. New England Journal of Medicine. 1998;**339**(10):659-666. DOI: 10.1056/NEJM199809033391003

[49] Sohns C, Zintl K, Zhao Y, et al. Impact of left ventricular function and heart failure symptoms on outcomes post ablation of atrial fibrillation in heart failure: CASTLE-AF Trial. Circulation. Arrhythmia and Electrophysiology. 2020;**13**(10):e008461. DOI: 10.1161/CIRCEP.120.008461

Section 2

Special Procedures in the Treatment of Atrial Fibrillation

Chapter 8

Left Atrial Appendage Occlusion: Current and Future

Dian Andina Munawar, Anggia Chairuddin Lubis and Muhammad Munawar

Abstract

Patients with non-valvular atrial fibrillation (NVAF) are at an increased risk of ischemic stroke due to the risks of thrombus formation. The left atrial appendage (LAA) is shown to be "the culprit" of thromboembolic events in NVAF and is currently a therapeutic target to prevent stroke. The absolute benefit of oral anticoagulation in the management of NVAF to improve cardiovascular outcomes has been well established. However, some patients are not good long-term candidates for oral anticoagulation for many reasons, including risks of bleeding, noncompliant to oral anticoagulation (OAC). Left atrial appendage occlusion (LAAO) provides an attractive alternative to reduce the risk of stroke for those who are contraindicated to OAC therapy.

Keywords: atrial fibrillation, left atrial appendage closure, left atrial appendage device, ischemic stroke, oral anticoagulation

1. Introduction

In patients with non-valvular atrial fibrillation (NVAF), oral anticoagulation (OAC) is part of mainstream therapy to prevent ischemic stroke [1], and the left atrial appendage (LAA) remains a focus of thrombus formation [2]. However, there are several situations that oral anticoagulation may be unsuitable, due to any individual history of major bleeding, personal risks of bleeding (e.g., fall risk in elderly or cerebral anomalies), noncompliant patients to OAC, or patients with high-risk occupation. Left atrial appendage occlusion (LAAO) has emerged as an alternative management to prevent stroke in NVAF patients who are not eligible for continuous OAC [3].

2. Left atrial appendage anatomy

The embryonic origin of LAA is different to atria. It is originated from the embryonic remnant of left atrium (LA) during first trimester, with a multilobed structure positioned anteriorly in the atrioventricular sulcus close to the left circumflex artery, the left phrenic nerve, and the left pulmonary veins [4]. The appendage contains numerous trabeculae, with a complex and highly variable anatomy. The LAA typically consists of three major components:

a. Ostium or "os," which defines its junction with body of the LA;

b. Lobar region, which is known to be the most variable anatomically. The difference of lobar region of LAA as seen by computed tomography angiography (CTA) is categorized into: (1) chicken wing; (2) cactus; (3) windsocks; and (4) cauliflower. It has been shown that the difference in the LAA morphology was independently associated with thromboembolic events [5, 6]. The first type of chicken-wing LAA can be a challenge for device implantation; [7] however, it has been associated with a lower stroke risk compared with the other three main morphologies described [8]. Multiple lobes with LAA greater than 40 mm will limit the use of certain devices. Deployment of LAAO device will be difficult for LAA with multiple lobes with branching close to ostium.

c. "Neck" is a narrow junction between the ostium, lobar region, and the landing zone for LAAO device. The size of the neck determines the applicability to use of certain occlude devices. The Watchman requires an equivalent implant depth and the device diameter. The Amplatzer device requires 10 mm space for deployment from the ostium [7].

3. Rationale for LAAO

Thromboembolic events in AF are correlated to loss of atrial contraction, stasis of blood flow, and thrombus formation, particularly in the LAA. The LAA is notoriously labeled as "human most lethal attachment," as it has been demonstrated that thrombus in the LAA is the primary source for thromboemboli [2]. A review of studies in patients with nonrheumatic heart disease demonstrated that 90% of LA thrombi examined by transesophageal echocardiography (TEE), cardiac surgery, or autopsy, were located in the LAA [9]. Another study also showed that LA thrombus was evident in 15% of patients without OAC after 48 hours of AF, in which almost all thrombi were found in LAA. The LAA is particularly prone to thrombus formation in AF due to its inherent anatomy with extensive trabeculations, increased blood stasis and hypercoagulability, and endothelial damage [10].

The role of the LAA as a source for thromboemboli in AF patients provides the rationale for ligation, amputation, or occlusion of the LAA structure, especially if patients are indicated for stroke prevention strategy; on the other hand, they are either contraindicated or noncompliant to long-term OAC. In addition, some LAAO techniques may have an additional role in sinus rhythm maintenance through non-pulmonary vein triggers elimination, atrial mass decrease, and atrial electrical remodeling reversion [11, 12].

4. Techniques for LAAO

Currently, there are two major different strategies in LAA exclusion from systemic circulation:

4.1 Surgical approach

The first reported resection of LAA in a human was by John Madden in 1949 [13]. In his report, he performed surgical excision of LAA structure during open

DOI: http://dx.doi.org/10.5772/intechopen.105776

heart surgery specifically aimed for stroke prevention in AF patients. This approach was not routinely done after this report was published. Nevertheless, LAA surgical closure is now class IIa indication in the 2020 American College of Cardiology (ACC)/American Heart Association (AHA) guidelines for management of patients with valvular heart disease undergoing heart surgery [14] and has currently become widely performed. Similarly, in patients with AF undergoing cardiac surgery, surgical LAA closure is also a class IIb indication based on 2019 ACC/AHA/Heart Rhythm Society (HRS) guidelines [15].

The method of LAA exclusion is usually dictated by the concomitant cardiosurgical procedure.

4.2 Percutaneous LAAO device

To date, several LAAO devices have been approved to be used worldwide (**Figure 1**).

4.2.1 Endocardial system

a. the Watchman (Boston Scientific, Natick, MA)

This device has been approved by the Federal Drug Administration (FDA) in the year of 2015 as an alternative to warfarin OAC based upon data from the PREVAIL and PROTECT-AF trials. The device system comprises of a 14 Fr (outer diameter), frame with fixation barbs, and fabric cover [16].

b. the Amplatzer Cardiac Plug/ACP (St. Jude Medical, St. Paul, MN)

The Amulet is a second-generation self-expanded LAAO. The device system includes 14.4–16.5 Fr delivery sheath, lobe and stabilization hook, and fixed-size cover disk [16].

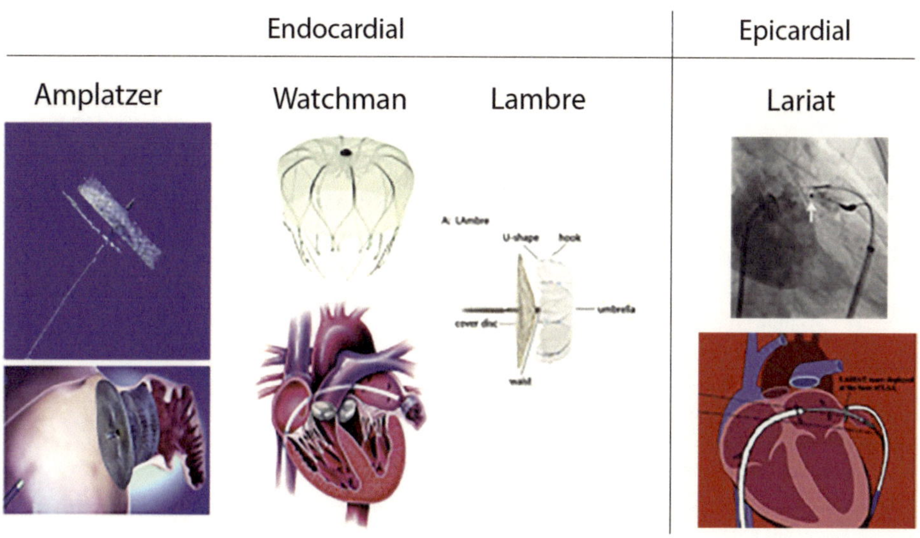

Figure 1.
LAAO devices (modified from [10, 16–18]).

c. LAmbreTM LAA Closure System (Lifetech Scientific Corporation)

LAmbre occluder is a Conformité Européenne (CE) recognized LAA closure device. It is a self-expanded device consisting of a 10.4–12.3 Fr sheath (delivery system), hook-embedded umbrella, and size adaptive cover [19]. In 2020, LAmbreTM LAA Closure System has obtained the approval by FDA for the commencement of an investigator-initiated clinical trial in the United States.

4.2.2 Epicardial system

a. the LARIAT suture delivery system (SentreHeart, Redwood City, CA)

The LARIAT device is a percutaneous epicardial ligation of the LAA. The device comprises of a snare with a pre-tied suture for LAA ligation, a 15-mm compliant occlusion balloon catheter, magnet-tipped guidewires, and a 12-F suture delivery device.

5. Indications and current recommendation

Indication for LAAO occlusion procedure is similar to standard indication of OAC in patients with AF. The need of OAC is justified by stroke risk factors that are summarized in the clinical risk-factor-based on established CHA_2DS_2-VASc score [Congestive heart failure, Hypertension, Age, Diabetes mellitus, Stroke, Vascular disease, and Sex category (female)]. However, when initiation of OAC strategy, individual potential risk of bleeding also needs to be assessed (**Table 1**).

Non-modifiable	Potentially modifiable	Modifiable	Biomarkers
• Age > 65 years • Previous major bleeding • Severe renal impairment (on dialysis or renal transplant) • Severe hepatic dysfunction (cirrhosis) • Malignancy • Genetic factors (e.g. CYP 2C9 polymorphisms) • Previous stroke, small-vessel disease, etc. • Diabetes mellitus • Cognitive impairment/ dementia	• Extreme frailty ± excessive risk of falls • Anemia • Reduced platelet count or function • Renal impairment with CrCl <60 mL/ min • VKA management strategy	• Hypertension/elevated SBP • Concomitant antiplatelet/ NSAID • Excessive alcohol intake • Non-adherence to OAC • Hazardous hobbies/ occupations • Bridging therapy with heparin • INR control (target 2.0–3.0), target TTR >70%c • Appropriate choice of OAC and • correct dosing	• GDF-15 • Cystatin C/ CKD-EPI • cTnT-hs • von Willebrand factor • other coagulation markers

CKD-EPI = Chronic Kidney Disease Epidemiology Collaboration; CrCl = creatinine clearance; cTnT-hs = high-sensitivity troponin T; CYP = cytochrome P; GDF-15 = growth differentiation factor-15; INR = international normalized ratio; NSAID = non-steroidal anti-inflammatory drug; OAC = oral anticoagulant; SBP = systolic blood pressure; TTR = time in therapeutic range; VKA = vitamin K antagonist.

Table 1.
Risk factors for bleeding with OAC and antiplatelet therapy (ESC guidelines 2020) [1].

	Source	COR	LOE	Recommendation
NVAF	2019 HRS [15]	IIB	B-NR	Percutaneous LAA occlusion may be considered in patients with AF at increased risk of stroke who have contraindications to long-term anticoagulation
VAF				No recommendation available

AF = atrial fibrillation; HRS = Heart Rhythm Society; LAA = Left atrial appendage; NR = Non-randomized; NVAF = Non-valvular atrial fibrillation; VAF = Valvular atrial fibrillation.

Table 2.
Current recommendation for percutaneous LAAO.

There are few absolute contraindications that potentially prevent some patients to have OAC as stroke prevention therapies. These include active major bleeding with unidentified and untreated source, comorbidities [e.g., severe anemia (Hb<80 g/L) or thrombocytopenia (<50 platelets/microliter)], or a high-risk bleeding episode such as intracranial hemorrhage. In such cases, non-drug options such as LAAO should be considered. Based on current existing guidelines, the recommendations of LAAO as stroke prevention option are:

5.1 Percutaneous approaches

Currently available recommendation for percutaneous LAAO is described in **Table 2**.

According to 2020 ESC guidelines for Atrial Fibrillation, recommendations for antithrombotic therapy after LAAO are mentioned in **Table 3** [1].

5.2 Surgical approaches

Table 4 shows current available recommendation for surgical LAA excision/occlusion approach.

Device/patient	Aspirin	OAC	Clopidogrel	Comments
Watchman/low bleeding risk	75–325 mg/day indefinitely by TOE	Start warfarin after procedure (target INR 2–3) until 45 days or continue until adequate LAA sealing is confirmed. NOAC is a possible alternative	Start 75 mg/day when OAC stopped, continue until 6 months after the procedure	Some centers do not withhold OAC at the time of procedure (no data to support/deny this approach)
Watchman/ high bleeding risk	75–325 mg/day indefinitely	None	75 mg/day for 1–6 months while ensuring adequate LAA sealing	Clopidogrel often given for shorter time in very high-risk situations
ACP/Amulet	75–325 mg/day indefinitely	None	75 mg/day for 1–6 months while ensuring adequate LAA sealing	Clopidogrel may replace long-term aspirin if better tolerated

ACP = Amplatzer Cardiac Plug; INR = international normalized ratio; LAA = Left atrial appendage; OAC = Oral anticoagulation; TOE = Transesophageal Echocardiography.

Table 3.
Anti-thrombotic recommendation after LAAO.

	Source	COR	LOE	Recommendation
NVAF	2019 HRS [15]	IIB	B-NR	Surgical occlusion of the LAA may be considered in patients with AF undergoing cardiac surgery, as a component of an overall heart team approach to the management of AF
VAF	2020 ACC/ AHA [14]	IIA	B-NR	For patients with AF or atrial flutter who are undergoing valve surgery, LA appendage ligation/excision is reasonable to reduce the risk of thromboembolic events
		IIA	B-NR	In patients undergoing LA surgical ablation of atrial arrhythmias and/or LA appendage ligation/excision, anticoagulation therapy is reasonable for at least 3 months after the procedure
VAF	2017 ESC [20]	IIB	B	Surgical excision or external clipping of the LA appendage may be considered in patients undergoing valve surgery
VHD	2020 ACC/ AHA [14]	III	B-NR	For patients without atrial arrhythmias who are undergoing valvular surgery, LA appendage occlusion/exclusion/amputation is potentially harmful

ACC = American College of Cardiology; AF = atrial fibrillation; AHA = American Heart association; ESC = European Society of Cardiology; HRS = Heart Rhythm Society; LA = Left atrium; LAA = Left atrial appendage; NR = Non-randomized; NVAF = Non-valvular atrial fibrillation; VAF = Valvular atrial fibrillation.

Table 4.
Current recommendation for surgical LAAO.

6. Post-procedural management and complications of percutaneous LAAO

6.1 Acute procedural-related complications

i. Access-related complications

The most common complication for percutaneous LAA closure is the risk of having vascular complications, including bleeding or hematoma in the groin, arteriovenous fistula, pseudoaneurysm, or retroperitoneal bleed. Some of these complications may require further intervention or blood transfusion. These risks are slightly higher than other interventional procedure, especially due to large delivery sheath used, and the procedure is commonly performed under oral anticoagulation [21]. Furthermore, frailty or tortuosity in the vascular anatomy is also very common in elderly patients [22].

ii. Transeptal access-related complications

There are few complications that can be related to transeptal access. Large delivery sheath for this procedure increases the risk of air embolism and subsequently increases the risk of stroke or myocardial infarction. In addition, transeptal puncture is also correlated with increased risk of pericardial effusion or tamponade that may require pericardiocentesis, with incidence of 1.39% [22, 23]. The risk of incidental aortic puncture from transeptal was also reported, which was closed by percutaneous approach with Amplatzer Septal Occluder [24].

iii. Device embolization

Due to anatomical variability of LAA, the risk of embolization of LAAO is higher. The incidence of LAA device embolization ranges between 0% and 2%. Recent reports suggest that The Amplatzer family of devices carries a higher risk of embolization as compared with the Watchman device, with incidence of 0.78% (3,585 patients) vs. 0.26% (7,236 patients)]; $p < 0.001$) [25]. Device embolization can be located either in the LA, left ventricle (LV), or aorta (Ao). Although the majority cases can be managed in semi-elective manner, some can be life-threatening and need emergency procedure. Limited data of secondary adverse events related to LAA device embolization such as mitral or aortic valve damage, LV outflow tract obstruction, cardiogenic shock, or death have been described [26]. Percutaneous retrieval is preferable as compared with surgical approach. Identification of the location of the embolized device is crucial to determine the retrieval strategy. Successful retrieval using percutaneous snare has been reported [27]. However, several complications such as iatrogenic aortic rupture requiring endovascular repair may occur [28].

iv. Other complication

Complications related to traumatic damage to surrounding structures (i.e., the circumflex coronary artery, pulmonary arteries, or pulmonary veins) have been previously described [29]. The NCDR registry showed that major complications, including in-hospital adverse events (2.16%), major bleeding (1.25%), were quite prevalent, whereas stroke (0.17%) and death (0.19%) were rare [23].

6.2 Long-term issues related to percutaneous LAAO

i. Iatrogenic atrial septal defects

Following transseptal LA access, iatrogenic atrial septal defects can be notable from either transthoracic or transesophageal echocardiogram. This complication can either disappear within 6 months after the procedure or persist in a small proportion of patients. Nevertheless, no hemodynamic consequences have been reported from this [30].

ii. Peri-device leakage

The target of LAAO procedure is to get a complete closure of the LAA in order to lower the risk of thromboembolism in AF patients. In the early experience of LAAO, peri-device leakage was quite prevalent. The PROTECT-AF study showed that approximately 32% of patients still have residual leak at 1 year after procedure. However, this did not seem to increase the risk of thromboembolism [31]. Furthermore, the incidence of this outcome has markedly reduced in the more recent registries, which ranging from 0.2 to1% [23, 32].

iii. Device-related thrombosis (DRT)

The main reasons of DRT remain unknown. It is postulated that the incidence of DRT is combination of either procedural factors (i.e., technique of implant or type of devices used), patient factors (i.e. patient frailty, LV dysfunction, or AF duration), or post-implant management factors (i.e., duration and type of antithrombotic therapies used) [33]. Few large studies of DRT for Watchman device such as the PROTECT AF, PREVAIL trials, CAP, and CAP2 evaluated procedural outcomes with TOE at 45 days and 12 months and at 6 months in the RCTs. Over 4 years of mean follow-up, it was demonstrated that the rate of DRT was 3.74%. The main characteristics of patients with DRT observed in this study are higher CHA2DS2VASc scores, permanent AF, and larger LAAs. The presence of DRT was also shown to be associated with a 3.55-fold increase rate of thromboembolic events [34].

7. Current evidence of short- and long-term outcomes after LAAO

The difficulties in managing patients with AF and high bleeding risk pursued a new approach of stroke prevention in AF patients. The first randomized study of LAAC with Watchman device, PROTECT AF [21], which was published in 2009, showed non-inferiority results as compared with standard warfarin therapy. This study randomized AF patients with a $CHADS_2$ score ≥ 1, to either Watchman implantation or OAC with warfarin. At 1.5 years of follow-up, it is shown that LAAC was equivalent for stroke prevention or all-cause mortality. The efficacy of LAA occlusion was also demonstrated in a longer-term follow-up of PROTECT AF trial. At a mean follow-up of 2.3 years, the primary efficacy endpoint is shown to be non-inferior for device [35].

Similar results were shown by the second randomized trial, PREVAIL (Evaluation of the WATCHMAN LAA Closure Device in Patients With Atrial Fibrillation Versus Long-Term Warfarin Therapy) [36]. The PREVAIL trial has given additional information to PROTECT AF trial by a Bayesian non-inferiority design approach. The study showed that LAAO with the Watchman device was not non-inferior to warfarin for the primary efficacy composite endpoint, including all-cause stroke, cardiovascular or unexplained death, and serious events (SE). In addition, LAAO was non-inferior to warfarin for the occurrence of late ischemic events after the first 7 days following randomization. Furthermore, the safety endpoint and successful rate of LAAO are high, even in the center with high numbers of limited experience operators of LAAO implantation within a higher-risk patient population.

In a long-term 5-year outcomes report from the PREVAIL trial and PROTECT AF trial [37], it was demonstrated that LAAC with the Watchman device provides a similar degree of stroke prevention in non-valvular AF patients to OAC with warfarin. Furthermore, with its ability to minimize major bleeding, particularly hemorrhagic stroke. LAAC results in less death than Warfarin [37].

The more recent randomized prospective, multicenter, randomized noninferiority study, PRAGUE-17, compared two treatment strategies in moderate to high-risk AF patients (i.e., patients with history of significant bleeding or history of cardiovascular event(s) or a with CHA2DS2VASc $\geq$3 and HAS-BLED score ≥ 2) [38]. This study randomized 402 patients with AF into percutaneous LAAC versus NOAC. After median follow-up of 3.5 year, LAAC was shown to be non-inferior to DOACs for the primary endpoint and the components of the composite endpoint, such as cardiovascular death, all-stroke/transient ischemic attack, clinically relevant bleeding, and for nonprocedural clinically relevant bleeding [39].

8. Conclusion

LAA is an important anatomic area that is involved in thrombus formation in the left atrium, which is also a determinant in the risk of thromboembolic events in patients with AF. LAAO procedure provides an important alternative to pharmacological strategy in AF patients, especially for patients with stroke prevention indication and contraindicated or noncompliant to oral anticoagulation. It is evident that LAAO is safe and effective with high implant success rate and improving complication rate. Long-term data regarding in the stroke outcomes as compared with standard strategy are necessary.

Author details

Dian Andina Munawar[1,2], Anggia Chairuddin Lubis[3] and Muhammad Munawar[1,2]*

1 Faculty of Medicine, Department of Cardiology and Vascular Medicine, Universitas Indonesia, Jakarta, Indonesia

2 Binawaluya Cardiac Centre, Jakarta, Indonesia

3 Department of Cardiology, Universitas Sumatera Utara, North Sumatera, Indonesia

*Address all correspondence to: muna286@gmail.com

References

[1] Hindricks G, Potpara T, Dagres N, Arbelo E, Bax JJ, Blomström-Lundqvist C, et al. ESC Guidelines for the diagnosis and management of atrial fibrillation developed in collaboration with the European Association for Cardio-Thoracic Surgery (EACTS): The Task Force for the diagnosis and management of atrial fibrillation of the European Society of Cardiology (ESC) Developed with the special contribution of the European Heart Rhythm Association (EHRA) of the ESC. European Heart Journal. 2020;**42**(5):373-498. DOI: 10.1093/eurheartj/ehaa612

[2] Johnson WD, Ganjoo AK, Stone CD, Srivyas RC, Howard M. The left atrial appendage: Our most lethal human attachment! Surgical implications. European Journal of Cardiothoracic Surgery. 2000;**17**(6):718-722. DOI: 10.1016/s1010-7940(00)00419-x

[3] Alkhouli M, Noseworthy PA, Rihal CS, Holmes DR Jr. Stroke prevention in nonvalvular atrial fibrillation: A stakeholder perspective. Journal of American College Cardiology. 2018;**71**(24):2790-2801. DOI: 10.1016/j.jacc.2018.04.013

[4] Al-Saady NM, Obel OA, Camm AJ. Left atrial appendage: Structure, function, and role in thromboembolism. Heart. 1999;**82**(5):547-554. DOI: 10.1136/hrt.82.5.547

[5] Khurram IM, Dewire J, Mager M, et al. Relationship between left atrial appendage morphology and stroke in patients with atrial fibrillation. Heart Rhythm. 2013;**10**(12):1843-1849. DOI: 10.1016/j.hrthm.2013.09.065

[6] Anselmino M, Scaglione M, Di Biase L, et al. Left atrial appendage morphology and silent cerebral ischemia in patients with atrial fibrillation. Heart Rhythm. 2014;**11**(1):2-7. DOI: 10.1016/j.hrthm.2013.10.020

[7] Don C, Cook A, Reisman M. LAA anatomy. In: Saw J, Kar S, Price M, editors. Left Atrial Appendage Closure: Mechanical Approached to Stroke Prevention in Atrial Fibrillation. Humana Press; Switzerland. 2016

[8] Di Biase L, Santangeli P, Anselmino M, et al. Does the left atrial appendage morphology correlate with the risk of stroke in patients with atrial fibrillation? Results from a multicenter study. Journal of American College of Cardiology. 2012;**60**(6):531-538. DOI: 10.1016/j.jacc.2012.04.032

[9] Blackshear JL, Odell JA. Appendage obliteration to reduce stroke in cardiac surgical patients with atrial fibrillation. The Annals of Thoracic Surgery. 1996;**61**(2):755-759. DOI: 10.1016/0003-4975(95)00887-x

[10] Lin AC, Knight BP. Left atrial appendage closure. Progress in Cardiovascular Diseases. 2015;**58**(2):195-201. DOI: 10.1016/j.pcad.2015.07.009

[11] Kawamura M, Scheinman MM, Lee RJ, Badhwar N. Left atrial appendage ligation in patients with atrial fibrillation leads to a decrease in atrial dispersion. Journal of American Heart Association. 2015;**4**(5):e001581

[12] Lakkireddy D, Sridhar Mahankali A, Kanmanthareddy A, et al. Left atrial appendage ligation and ablation for persistent atrial fibrillation: The LAALA-AF Registry. JACC Clinical Electrophysiology. 2015;**1**(3):153-160. DOI: 10.1016/j.jacep.2015.04.006

[13] Madden JL. Resection of the left auricular appendix; a prophylaxis for recurrent arterial emboli. Journal of American Medical Association. 1949;**140**(9):769-772. DOI: 10.1001/jama.1949.02900440011003

[14] Otto CM, Nishimura RA, Bonow RO, Carabello BA, Erwin JP, 3rd, Gentile F, et al. ACC/AHA Guideline for the Management of Patients With Valvular Heart Disease: Executive Summary: A Report of the American College of Cardiology/American Heart Association Joint Committee on Clinical Practice Guidelines. Circulation. 2021;**143**(5):e35-e71. DOI: 10.1161/CIR.0000000000000932

[15] Writing Group M, January CT, Wann LS, Calkins H, Chen LY, Cigarroa JE, et al. AHA/ACC/HRS focused update of the 2014 AHA/ACC/HRS guideline for the management of patients with atrial fibrillation: A Report of the American College of Cardiology/American Heart Association Task Force on Clinical Practice Guidelines and the Heart Rhythm Society. Heart Rhythm. 2019;**16**(8):e66-e93. DOI: 10.1016/j.hrthm.2019.01.024

[16] Chen S, Chun KRJ, Bordignon S, et al. Left atrial appendage occlusion using LAmbre Amulet and Watchman in atrial fibrillation. Journal of Cardiology. 2019;**73**(4):299-306. DOI: 10.1016/j.jjcc.2018.10.010

[17] Dar T, Turagam MK, Yarlagadda B, Tantary M, Sheldon SH, Lakkireddy D. Indication, patient selection, and referral pathways for left atrial appendage closure. Intervention Cardiology Clinics. 2018;**7**(2):169-183. DOI: 10.1016/j.iccl.2017.12.003

[18] Srivastava MC, See VY, Dawood MY, Price MJ. A review of the LARIAT device: Insights from the cumulative clinical experience. Springerplus. 2015;**4**:522. DOI: 10.1186/s40064-015-1289-8

[19] Chen S, Schmidt B, Bordignon S, et al. Feasibility of percutaneous left atrial appendage closure using a novel LAmbre occluder in patients with atrial fibrillation: Initial results from a prospective cohort registry study. Journal of Cardiovascular Electrophysiology. 2018;**29**(2):291-297. DOI: 10.1111/jce.13385

[20] Baumgartner H, Falk V, Bax JJ, De Bonis M, Hamm C, Holm PJ, et al. ESC/EACTS Guidelines for the management of valvular heart disease. European Heart Journal. 2017;**38**(36):2739-2791. DOI: 10.1093/eurheartj/ehx391

[21] Holmes DR, Reddy VY, Turi ZG, et al. Percutaneous closure of the left atrial appendage versus warfarin therapy for prevention of stroke in patients with atrial fibrillation: A randomised non-inferiority trial. Lancet. 2009;**374**(9689):534-542

[22] Perrotta L, Bordignon S, Dugo D, et al. Complications from left atrial appendage exclusion devices. Journal of Atrial Fibrillation. 2014;7(1):1034-1034. DOI: 10.4022/jafib.1034

[23] Freeman JV, Varosy P, Price MJ, et al. The NCDR left atrial appendage occlusion registry. Journal of American College of Cardiology. 2020;**75**(13):1503-1518. DOI: 10.1016/j.jacc.2019.12.040

[24] Hartono, B., et al. "Amplatzer septal occluder sealed the complicating aortic root perforation during transseptal procedure." JACC Cardiovasc Interv 2012;**5**(4):450-451

[25] Asmarats L, Rodes-Cabau J. Percutaneous left atrial appendage closure: Current devices and clinical outcomes. Circulation of Cardiovascular Intervention. 2017 Nov;**10**(11):e005359.

[26] Jazayeri MA, Vuddanda V, Turagam MK, et al. Safety profiles of percutaneous left atrial appendage closure devices: An analysis of the Food and Drug Administration Manufacturer and User Facility Device Experience (MAUDE) database from 2009 to 2016. Journal of Cardiovascular Electrophysiology. 2018;**29**(1):5-13. DOI: 10.1111/jce.13362

[27] Lubis AC, Iqbal M, Munawar DA, Hartono B, Munawar M. A simple percutaneous retrieval technique for an embolized watchman left atrial appendage closure device in the thoracic aorta using a homemade snare. International Heart Journal. 2021;**62**(5):1153-1155

[28] Mastrangelo A, Galli S, Montorsi P, Bartorelli AL. Aortic rupture and hemorrhagic shock after percutaneous retrieval of an embolized left atrial appendage occluder. JACC Case Reports. 2022;**4**(8):486-490. DOI: 10.1016/j.jaccas.2022.03.004

[29] Sepahpour A, Ng MK, Storey P, McGuire MA. Death from pulmonary artery erosion complicating implantation of percutaneous left atrial appendage occlusion device. Heart Rhythm. 2013;**10**(12):1810-1811. DOI: 10.1016/j.hrthm.2013.07.046

[30] Onalan O, Crystal E. Left atrial appendage exclusion for stroke prevention in patients with nonrheumatic atrial fibrillation. Stroke. 2007;**38**(2 Suppl):624-630. DOI: 10.1161/01.Str.0000250166.06949.95

[31] Viles-Gonzalez JF, Kar S, Douglas P, et al. The clinical impact of incomplete left atrial appendage closure with the Watchman Device in patients with atrial fibrillation: A PROTECT AF (Percutaneous Closure of the Left Atrial Appendage Versus Warfarin Therapy for Prevention of Stroke in Patients With Atrial Fibrillation) substudy. Journal of American College of Cardiology. 2012;**59**(10):923-929. DOI: 10.1016/j.jacc.2011.11.028

[32] Boersma LV, Ince H, Kische S, et al. Evaluating Real-World Clinical Outcomes in Atrial Fibrillation Patients Receiving the WATCHMAN Left Atrial Appendage Closure Technology: Final 2-Year Outcome Data of the EWOLUTION Trial Focusing on History of Stroke and Hemorrhage. Circulation. Arrhythmia and Electrophysiology. 2019;**12**(4):e006841. DOI: 10.1161/circep.118.006841

[33] Alfadhel M, Nestelberger T, Samuel R, McAlister C, Saw J. Left atrial appendage closure – Current status and future directions. Progress in Cardiovascular Diseases. 2021;**69**:101-109. DOI: 10.1016/j.pcad.2021.11.013

[34] Dukkipati SR, Kar S, Holmes DR, et al. Device-related thrombus after left atrial appendage closure: Incidence, predictors, and outcomes. Circulation. 2018;**138**(9):874-885. DOI: 10.1161/CIRCULATIONAHA.118.035090

[35] Reddy VY, Doshi SK, Sievert H, et al. Percutaneous left atrial appendage closure for stroke prophylaxis in patients with atrial fibrillation: 2.3-Year Follow-up of the PROTECT AF (Watchman Left Atrial Appendage System for Embolic Protection in Patients with Atrial Fibrillation) Trial. Circulation. 2013;**127**(6):720-729

[36] Holmes DR Jr, Kar S, Price MJ, et al. Prospective randomized evaluation of the Watchman Left Atrial Appendage Closure device in patients with atrial fibrillation versus long-term warfarin therapy: The PREVAIL trial. Journal of American Colege of Cardiology. 2014;**64**(1):1-12. DOI: 10.1016/j.jacc.2014.04.029

[37] Reddy VY, Doshi SK, Kar S, et al. 5-year outcomes after left atrial appendage closure: From the PREVAIL and PROTECT AF Trials. Journal of American Colege of Cardiology. 2017;**70**(24):2964-2975

[38] Osmancik P, Tousek P, Herman D, et al. Interventional left atrial appendage closure vs novel anticoagulation agents in patients with atrial fibrillation indicated for long-term anticoagulation (PRAGUE-17 study). American Heart Journal. 2017;**183**:108-114. DOI: 10.1016/j.ahj.2016.10.003

[39] Osmancik P, Herman D, Neuzil P, et al. 4-year outcomes after left atrial appendage closure versus Nonwarfarin oral anticoagulation for atrial fibrillation. Journal of American College of Cardiology. 2022;**79**(1):1-14. DOI: 10.1016/j.jacc.2021.10.023

Chapter 9

Vein of Marshall Ethanol Infusion in Setting of Atrial Fibrillation Ablation

Andrea Rossi, Procolo Marchese and Marcello Piacenti

Abstract

Catheter ablation especially in persistent atrial fibrillation has limited success. Strategies beyond pulmonary veins isolation failed to demonstrate improvement of long-term rhythm maintenance. The vein of Marshall (VOM) is a promising therapeutic target as it fit perfectly with "Coumel's triangle": triggers in form of focal activities or stable reentries priming atrial fibrillation comes typically from tissue surrounding the VOM, it colocalize with mitral line especially in the epicardial part difficult to approach by endocardial ablations, it contains autonomic parasympathetic and sympathetic innervation implicated in arrhythmogenesis. Epicardial chemical ablation by ethanol delivery directly inside the vein of Marshall represents an attractive therapeutic approach eliminating arrhythmic triggers and autonomic modulators and, as it colocalize with the trajectory of the mitral isthmus, completing the integrity of that linear lesion. Based on advantages provided from VOM alcoholization, this technique has been progressively introduced in addiction to standard ablation strategies in atrial fibrillation treatment. This chapter aims to describe the electrophysiological characteristics of vein of Marshall, the technical aspects of ethanol delivery and the evidences from the literature supporting the emerging role of VOM alcoholization in atrial fibrillation treatment.

Keywords: vein of Marshall, alcoholization, VOM-ETHO, atrial fibrillation, ablation

1. Introduction

Experimental and clinical studies have demonstrated that atrial myocardial tissue surrounding the vein of Marshall (VOM) can support electrical focal activities [1] or stable reentries [2] priming atrial fibrillation or synchronized atrial arrhythmias. Moreover, the epicardial region along the path of VOM contains autonomic parasympathetic [3, 4] and sympathetic [5] innervation that have been implicated in triggering AF [6] unveiling important technical issues in the treatment of this arrhythmia and in the maintenance of sinus rhythm after ablation procedures. Thus, VOM is a promising therapeutic target because it fits perfectly with Coumel's triangle components (trigger, substrate and autonomic tone). Since it is insulated by epicardial fat, physical ablation of the VOM bundle by radiofrequency has been highly challenging and potentially harmful. Chemical ablation by retrograde ethanol infusion in the Marshall vein (VOM-ETHO) has provided a new attractive approach for an efficient elimination of triggered activity originating from this region. As the atrial tissue surrounding the VOM connects the mitral annulus (coronary sinus) to the posterior left atrium (as well as the lateral ridge), this technique has proved to be highly effective in determining a complete mitral isthmus block both in terms of acute success and lesion durability [7].

2. Anatomical considerations

Embryologically, the VOM is a remnant of the left superior vena cava, which, as it becomes atretic during fetal growth, may remain open in form of small vein diramation draining into the coronary sinus [5]. In 1850 Marshall first described this venous structure draining into the coronary sinus with trajectory directed toward the lateral and posterior wall of left atrium and directed up to the left pulmonary veins [8]. The VOM descends obliquely, posterior to the left atrial (appendage (LAA) on the epicardial aspect of the LA lateral ridge, running along the postero-lateral LA toward the CS. A comprehensive study of the atrial venous anatomy is provided by Valderrabano and colleagues based on analysis of a series of VOM-ETHO procedures performed on a large population of 218 patients scheduled for atrial fibrillation ablation interventions [9]. In this research, beyond the VOM, that was the most commonly cannulated vein, other atrial veins were variably opacified by dye infusion through collateral flow. A consistent pattern of atrial branches arising from coronary ostium were observed (as depicted in **Figure 1**): septal vein, a second inferior vein, the VOM, LAA veins, anterior roof veins. Other veins not connected to the CS were detected such as roof veins commonly connected with posterior veins and extracardiac collaterals.

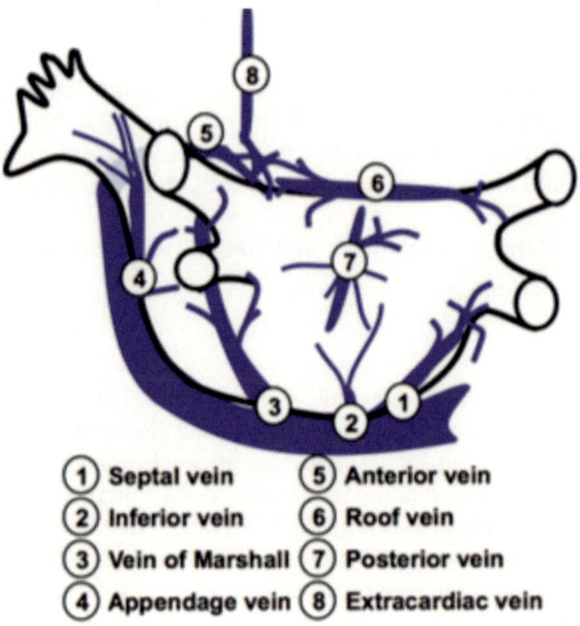

Figure 1.
Diagrammatic representation of atrial venous circulation from the posterior aspect of the left atrium. From: Valderrabano et al. [9].

VOM is typically localized at the ostial aspect of the valve of Vieussens. The incidence of VOM identification is about 75–92% according to data in the literature [9, 10]. Distance between CS ostium and VOM is 4.25 ± 2.57 cm, with substantial variability. VOM length before branching was 2.99 ± 1.82 cm. VOM is typically a true atrial vein, with branches and visible venules draining the neighboring atrial tissue. Variable branching was present in 78.2% of cases. According to relation to the left inferior pulmonary vein, VOM presents variable trajectory: smaller VOM which terminates before reaching the left inferior PV (17.6%), VOM visible up to the left inferior pulmonary vein (72.8%), VOM can reach the left superior pulmonary vein (9.6%). Communication between VOM and left pulmonary veins was demonstrated by contrast drainage in the left PVs during the VOM venogram, appearing to connect through the left pulmonary vein carina (it happens in 37.7% of cases).

3. VOM-ETHO procedure

The technique was pioneered by Valderrabano and coworkers in 2009 [11]. The protocol was studied in 17 dogs. VOM was visualized in 13. The electroanatomical map of left atrium repeated after ethanol infusion demonstrated a new crescent-shaped scar extending from mitral annulus in the posterior wall toward left pulmonary veins. To test the feasibility of VOM-ETHO in humans, 6 patients undergoing pulmonary veins antral isolation, had successful VOM cannulation and ethanol infusion with the confirmation of a new scar formation involving the infero-posterior left atrial wall extending toward the left pulmonary veins.

A right jugular approach [11–14] and femoral vein approach [15] have been described for VOM cannulation and alcohol delivery. There are reports of success rate of 74% (23 out 31 patients) for VOM venogram using the right jugular approach and 89% (17 out 19 patients) using the femoral approach. Valderrabano et al. reported that 86% (188 of 218) of the VOM was accessible using a right jugular approach with a LIMA angiographic catheter [16].

The technique for VOM cannulation and ethanol infusion was subsequently well reported by the Bordeaux group [17] demonstrating a high success rate of VOM cannulation of 92.6% (50 of 54) with a femoral approach using the LIMA (left internal mammary artery) catheter (**Figure 2**).

3.1 A step-by-step list actions

- from the right femoral vein, a steerable long sheat (Agilis NxT; Abbott) or long fixed curve sheath was inserted into the CS, guided by ablation catheter or steerable catheter. Once the long sheath was in place, a CS venogram was acquired (**Figure 3**, panel 1).

- A selective venogram of the VOM was performed using a 5-Fr angiography catheter (left internal mammary artery [LIMA] via the long sheat). To acquire a clearer venogram of the VOM and avoid the overlapping CS, a right anterior oblique (RAO) view was preferred (**Figure 3**, panel 2). The LIMA catheter was inserted into the CS point both posteriorly and superiorly in the RAO view. In addition, the contrast indentation indicating the location of the valve of Vieussens was carefully explored to find the ostium of VOM. At each location, a small amount of the contrast was injected through the LIMA catheter to confirm

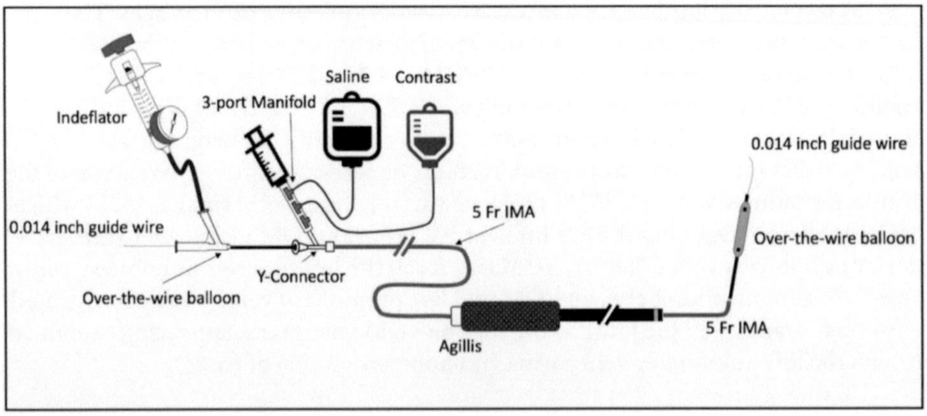

Figure 2.
A comprehensive schematic representation of the technical setting for ethanol infusion in the VOM. From Kitamura et al. [17].

engaging the VOM. When the VOM was not identified, a balloon occlusion venogram of CS was performed to explore the VOM.

- After engaging VOM by LIMA catheter, an angioplasty wire 0.014 inch supported by an over-the-wire balloon catheter was advanced into the VOM. An appropriate size of balloon (1.5–2.5 mm diameter and 6–15 mm length) was used depending on the size of the VOM (**Figure 3**, panel 3–4)

- The balloon was started to be inflated at low pressure (1–2 atm) until the operator feel some resistance on the inflator with a maximum of 6–8 atm in the VOM. After the balloon was inflated completely, the wire was removed.

- A selective venogram of the VOM was obtained by injecting 1 mL of contrast medium through the wire port of the balloon (**Figure 3**, panel 5)

- After confirming balloon occlusion and VOM distribution, 0.5–3 mL of ethanol (96% ethanol 10 mL) was slowly injected over 1 minute and selective venography of the VOM was repeated (**Figure 3**, panel 6–8). A total of 6 to 12 mL of ethanol was used as a maximum dose.

3.2 Tissue Ablation by VOM-ETHO

Ethanol infusion in the VOM leads to generation of a new low-voltage area posterior and superior to the coronary sinus, encompassing variable extents of the posterior left atrial wall and the anterior aspect of the left inferior pulmonary vein. The area of the scarring depends on the size of the VOM. Valderrabano et al. reported that the area of scar (bipolar voltage amplitude <0.5 mV) was 10.2 + – 5.7 cm^2 (range, 3.3 to 15.3 cm^2) in the first human experience.[17] On large population of over 700 patients, the Bordeaux group reported a scarring area of 10.2 + –5.3 cm^2 [10, 17]. In this experience factors contributing to reduction of VOM-ETHO effectiveness in lesion formation were: VOM dissection (10.7%), iodine leakage (3.0%), and VOM morphology without visible branches (3.0%). Ethanol infusion in a wrong vein was associated with less mitral line block (72.7% versus 95.8%, P = 0.012).

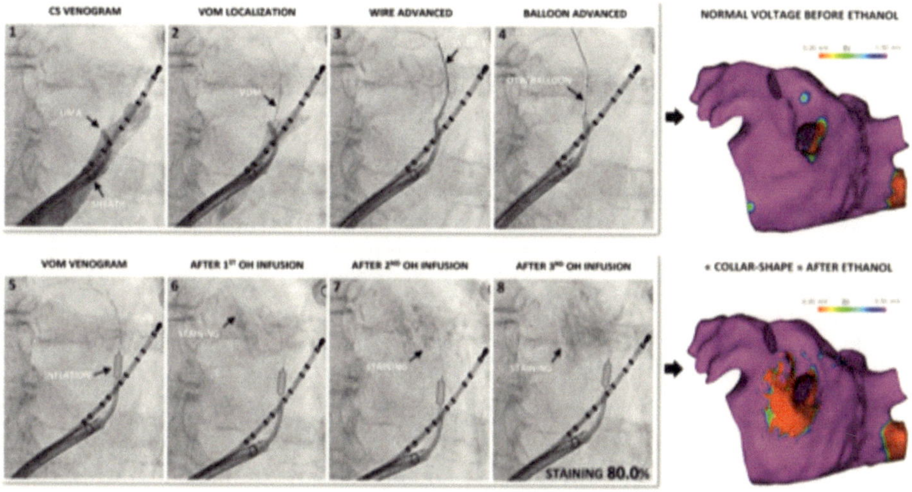

Figure 3.
Step-by-step actions for VOM cannulation and ethanol delivery (right panels). Left panels: Pre and post-VOM-ETHO bipolar maps indicating typical location and shaping of scarring formation. From: Kitamura et al. [17].

3.3 Technical issues and considerations

VOM-ETHO is highly feasible with a success rate of 91% from latest data on a population of over 700 patients [10]. Factors associated to procedural failure were: nonidentification of VOM (6.2%), noncannulation (1.5%) or ethanol infusion in the wrong vein (1.7%). The Vieussens valve was a helpful landmark and was visible in 63.2% of cases. Remarkably, previous ablation inside the coronary sinus was strictly associated to VOM nonidentification. The success rate of VOM-ETHO procedures increases with the experience of operators.

3.4 Complications

Complications related to VOM-ETHO procedures are reported in **Table 1**.

Acute and delayed pericardial effusion represented the most described complications. During the procedure, pericardial tamponade was generally due to inadvertent CS perforation during VOM cannulation maneuvers or steam pops occurred during ablation. After the procedure, subacute pericardial effusion requiring pericardiocentesis was related to inflammatory reaction after alcohol delivery. The higher rate of delayed cardiac effusion or tamponade observed in patients with VOM perforation advocates a causal relationship between the inflammatory reaction and the inadvertent drainage of ethanol in the pericardial space. LAA isolation occurring after VOM-ETHO procedures may be observed in patients with previous extensive ablation settings involving septal and anterior scarring.

4. Role of VOM Bundle in atrial tachycardias

Atrial tachycardias (ATs) are often seen in the context of atrial fibrillation ablation implicating macroreentrant or scar-related mechanisms [19, 20].

Event	Rate (%)	Time	Comment	Management
VOM perforation	2.8	Acute	Infusion still feasible but with higher risk of delayed tamponade	Anti-inflammatory drugs and repeated echocardiography
pericarditis	1.8	Delayed	Usually at day 2	anti-inflammatory drugs
Delayed tamponade	0.8–6	Delayed	serous nature of cardiac effusion in ⅔ of patients. Usually due to inflammatory reaction	pericardiocentesis
Stroke	0.6–1	Delayed	stroke rate in the reported range	medical management
Acute tamponade	0.1–0.2	Acute	related to cannulation manoeuvers and eventual per-procedural stem pops	Surgical drainage necessary
Anaphylaxis	<0.2	Acute	generally in case of hemodynamic collapse during infusion	adrenaline, corticosteroids
High Degree AVB	<0.2	Acute	must be favored by very proximal VOM ostium	monitoring AV conduction during ethanol infusion
LAA Isolation	0.2	Acute	risk increased in case of large anterior scarring	Bachmann conduction assessment prior to VOM-ETHO in case of history of previous extensive ablations

Modified from: Kamakura et al. [10]; and Valderrábano et al. [18].

Table 1.
Complications rate during VOM-ETHO procedures.

Radiofrequency catheter ablation is an effective therapy for patients with AF but perimitral ATs and localized reentry circuits commonly appear after pulmonary vein isolation or additional linear lesion in the left atrium [21]. Patients having connections between Marshall bundle and the myocardium of coronary sinus, left atrium or pulmonary veins, may develop the anatomical substrate to generate localized reentry circuits or macroreentrant ATs around the mitral isthmus, using the epicardial Marshall bundle [22]. Vlachos et al. [23], considering a population of 140 patients previously underwent a pulmonary vein isolation procedure, reported that the Marshall bundle is involved in a higher proportion of post-AF ablation ATs (30.2%), being 51.7% macroreentrant ATs and 48.3% localized reentry. Marshall bundle-dependent ATs can be terminated with RF ablation, either endocardial via Marshall-bundle-left atrium connection, or epicardially via Marshall bundle-CS connections, and with ethanol infusion inside the VOM being the Marshall bundle an electrically protected, isolated anatomical structure, difficult to target with RF ablation (**Figures 4** and 5) [24].

Endocardial ablation from within the left atrium may not successfully ablate the Marshall bundle, owing to the distance from endocardium to the critical site. As RF ablation induces a tissue heating by mostly resistive mechanism, the difficult to reach the epicardial Marshall bundle may explain the high failure rate of mitral isthmus block in published studies [25, 26]. For these reasons ethanol infusion inside the VOM

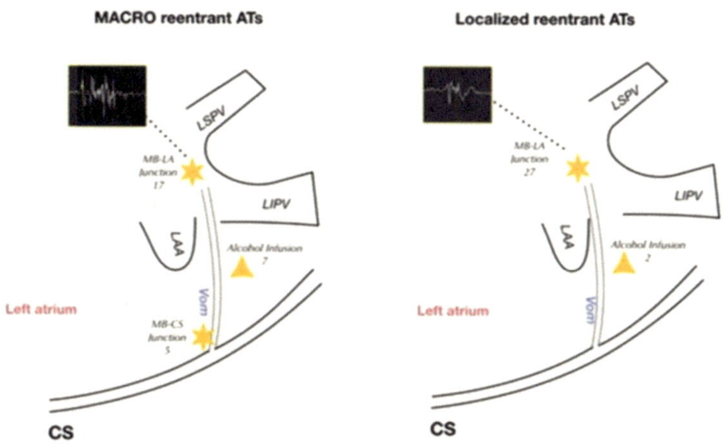

Figure 4.
The bipolar EGMs recorded in MB-LA connections and MB-CS connections have a characteristic electrophysiological pattern: high-frequency long-duration amplitude multicomponent (multiphasic) EGMs. From Vlachos et al. [2].

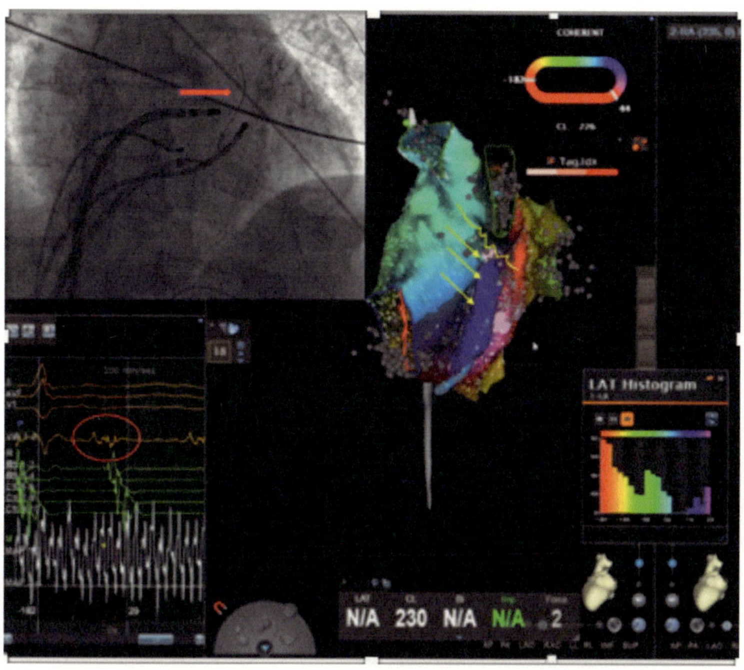

Figure 5.
Example of Marshall Bundle-related perimitral circuit in a patient with previous pulmonary vein isolation and linear lesions in the left atrium (mitral line and roofline). Note that part of the circuit is lacking during endocardial mapping on the LAT Histogram (CARTO7 module). Circuit mapping is completed by annotating signals recorded on Vision-Wire (red arrow) in the VOM. Diastolic signal recorded on the mapping wire placed in the VOM appears fragmented and of long duration.

may represent an adjunctive standalone strategy in patients with refractory Marshall bundle-related perimitral ATs or localized reentry circuits [14, 27, 28]. The additional use of VOM-ETHO strategy seems to improve ablation rates when compared with RF ablation alone [25, 26].

5. VOM-ETHO in setting of atrial fibrillation. Randomized clinical trials

The VENUS-AF Trial (Vein of Marshall EthaNol in Untreated perSistent) completed in 2018 and published in 2020 [18], was a multicenter, randomized clinical trial comparing the rhythm-control effectiveness of 2 ablation strategies: catheter ablation alone or combined with vein of Marshall ethanol infusion in de novo ablation of AF in a 1:1.15 fashion (including 15% more patients in the VOM group predicting a 15% failure to complete the VOM procedure thus being able to compare VOM-completed patients with controls in a 1:1 ratio). Patients were recruited from 12 referral centers in the United States and were eligible if they were between 18 and 85 years of age and had symptomatic persistent AF (sustained AF lasting >7 days) refractory to at least 1 antiarrhythmic agent. Exclusion criteria included previous AF ablation attempts and left atrial diameter or volume exceeding 65 mm or 200 mL, respectively. The primary endpoint was freedom from AF or AT 30-second duration over 1-year follow-up, with 1-months continuous monitoring at 6 and 12 months, after a single procedure. A total of 343 patients were enrolled (185 randomized to VOM and 158 to PVI). VOM-ETHO was successfully completed in 155 of 185 patients. After a single procedure, 49.2% (91/185) in the VOM group resulted free from AT/AF compared to 38% (60/185) in the PVI group (p = 0.04). Considering patients with VOM-ETHO procedure successfully completed (as-treated analysis), the primary outcome was reached in 80/115 patients in the VOM group (51.6%, p = 0.02). Notably, AF burden, freedom from AF after multiple procedures and mitral line block achievement were significantly improved in VOM-treated patients. Kaplan–Meier plots showed significant reduction in AF or AT recurrence in the VOM group, in both the as-randomized analysis (hazard ratio 0.73; 95% CI 0.53–1.00; P 5 0.05) and the as-treated analysis (hazard ratio 0.67; 95% CI 0.47–0.93; P 5 0.02) (**Figure 6**). Interestingly, considering subjects with mitral line bidirectional block achievement, patients randomized to VOM-ETHO group (75 of 138) showed a better outcome respect to patients randomized to "ablation only" group (30 of 81) in terms of freedom from AT/AF in 1 year follow-up (54.3% vs. 37%, OR 0.49; 95% CI 0.28–0.87; P 5 0.01) [29].

Marshall-PLAN trial from the Bordeaux group adopted VOM-ETHO added to routine workflow in AF catheter ablation. Marshall-PLAN (Marshall bundle elimination, Pulmonary vein isolation, and Line completion for ANatomical ablation) trial [30] prospectively enrolled 75 consecutive patients with persistent AF for a de novo ablation procedure. All patients underwent VOM-ETHO and coronary sinus

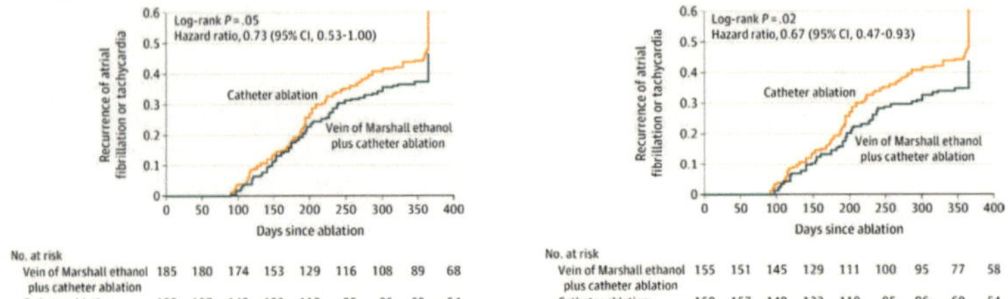

Figure 6.
Outcomes of the VENUS trial. A: time-to-recurrence of atrial fibrillation/atrial tachycardia "as randomized". B: time to recurrence excluding patients "as-treated", excluding patients in whom VOM-ETHO procedure was not completed. From: Valderrábano et al. [18].

musculature ablation, PVI and anatomical isthmuses linear ablation (mitral, roof and cavotricuspid isthmus) (**Figure 7**). The primary endpoint was 12-months freedom from AF/atrial tachycardia. VOM-ETHO was completed in 69 patients (92%). The full lesion set was successfully completed in 68 patients (91%). At 12 months, 54 of 75 patients (72%) were free from AF/AT after a single procedure (without antiarrhythmic drugs) in the overall cohort. In the subset of patients with a complete lesion set (VOM-ETHO and anatomical lines), the single procedure success rate was 79%. After 1 or 2 procedures, 67 of 75 patients (89%) remained free from AF/AT without antiarrhythmic drugs (**Figure 8**).

In the Marshall-PLAN trial anatomical structures considered critical to the fibrillatory process were targeted (PVs, CS and Marshall bundle network). VOM ethanol infusion was central to the Marshall-PLAN as it enhances the success of subsequent

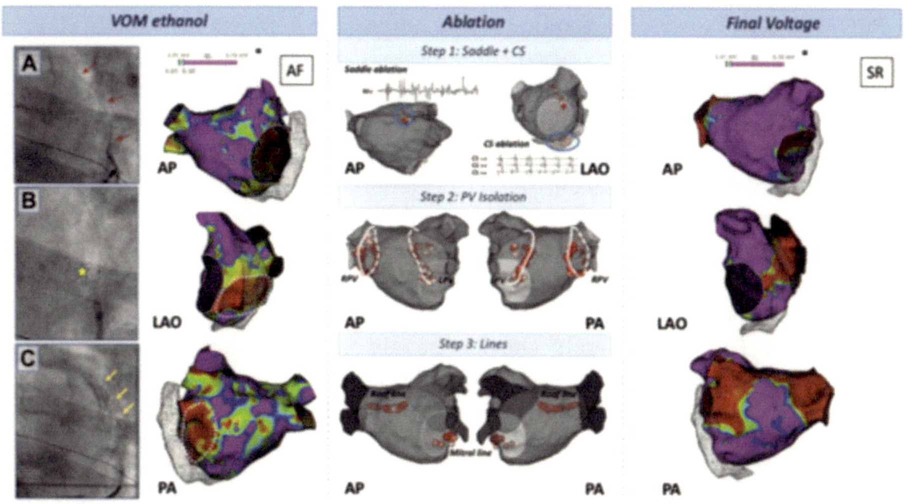

Figure 7.
Marshall-PLAN lesion set. Left: steps for ethanol infusion into vein of Marshall (VOM); A: contrast injection into the VOM with evidence of vein arborization (red arrows). B: (insertion of the angioplasty balloon inflated in the proximal portion of the VOM (yellow star: radiopaque marker of balloon). C: contrast injection in the VOM after alcoholization shows contrast staining. Middle: ablation set in the LA: targeting of CS musculature and "saddle" confirmed by fractionated local electrograms, pulmonary veins isolation and anatomical lines for roof and mitral isthmuses. Right: LA voltage map in sinus rhythm showing final lesion set. From: Derval et al. [30].

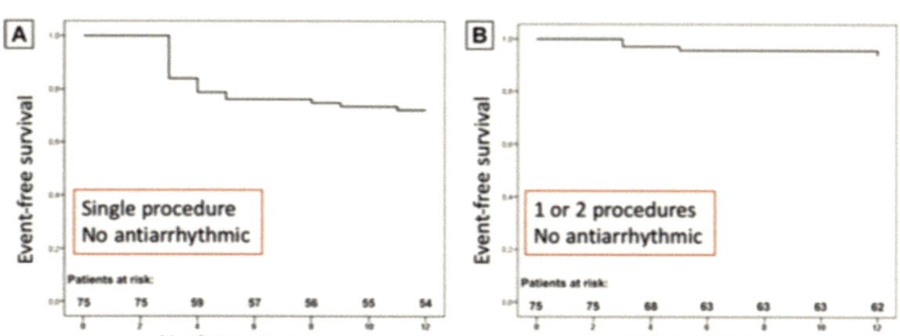

Figure 8.
Freedom from atrial fibrillation (AF)/Atrial tachycardia (AT)-Kaplan–Meier event-free survival curves after a single ablation procedure, without antiarrhythmic drugs (A), and after 1 or 2 procedures, without antiarrhythmic drugs (B). From Derval et al. [30].

PVI and linear ablation. Patients experiencing AF/AT recurrences after the first procedure demonstrated gaps in the original lesion set. Interestingly, anatomical sites of gaps were clustered in the right posterior carina/roofline and mitral line. Reconnections was not related to conduction recovery through the VOM but rather due to reconnections at the CS/LA interface. These findings suggest that other epicardial structures could play important roles in achieving durable transmural lesions, such as the septopulmonary bundle (for right PVs and roof line), the CS (for the mitral line), and the CTI. It is important to note that patients with incomplete lesion set at the index procedures had arrhythmic recurrences. In the Marshall-PLAN trial two patients experienced a transient ischaemic attack with no neurologic sequelae and four patients had post-ablation pericarditis. Three patients experienced minor groin hematoma.

In terms of LA function, the analysis of A-wave velocities suggested significant improvements in LA function at 12 months in patients without arrhythmic recurrences after the index procedure.

PROMPT-AF (Prospective Randomized Comparison between upgraded "2C3L" vs. PVI approach for the catheter ablation of persistent atrial fibrillation) [31] aimed to compare VOM-ETHO added to PVI plus roofline, mitral line and CTI ablation to PVI alone with randomized design. Unlike the original project, the study published in 2021 [32] does not have a randomized design and enrolled 191 patients who underwent their first catheter ablation of persistent atrial fibrillation (PeAF). The 2C3L technique is a fixed ablation approach consisting of bilateral circumferential PVI and three linear ablation lesion sets across the mitral isthmus, left atrial roof, and cavo-tricuspid isthmus. Patients were selected consecutively and compared for VOM-ETHO plus 2C3L approach (group 1) and 2C3L approach "RF only" (group 2). The follow-up duration was 12 months. The primary endpoint was the rate of documented atrial arrhythmias lasting >30 seconds without any antiarrhythmic drugs, in 12 months after index ablation procedures considering a blanking period of 3 months. The final population consisted of 191 patients (66 in the group 1 and 125 in the group 2). Successful VOM-ETHO was performed in 53 patients in group 1 (VOM not cannulated in 12, VOM dissection in one). At the index procedure, 100% of patients showed successful PVI, bidirectional roofline block and CTI block while mitral isthmus block was achieved in 95.5% of patients in group 1 and 80.8% in group 2 (p 0.006). At 12-months follow-up, 58 (87.9%) patients were free from AF/AT in group 1 compared with 81 (64.8%) in group 2 ($p < 0.001$) (2 in group 1 and 3 in group 2 patients were on AAD during the 12-months follow-up). Considering patients who received successful VOM-ETHO (53), freedom from AF/AT was achieved in 47 (88.7%). At the survival analysis, group 1 showed higher survival freedom from AT recurrence after adjustment for age, LA diameter, long-standing persistent atrial fibrillation, hypertension, and heart failure (HR 0.27, 95% CI 0.12–0.59) (**Figure 9**). Two patient experienced mild complication in the "VOM-ETHO" group: one mild pericardial effusion with self-relief and one fluid overload during the procedure. Eight complications occurred in seven (5.6%) patients in "ablation only" group including four fluid overload, one mild pericardial effusion with self-relief, two arteriovenous fistulae, and one pleural effusion. No severe complications like death, stroke or atrial-esophageal fistula were observed.

6. Conclusions

Retrograde ethanol alcoholization of the vein of Marshall (VOM-ETHO) is a feasible, safe and effective strategy in treating atrial tachycardias depending on the

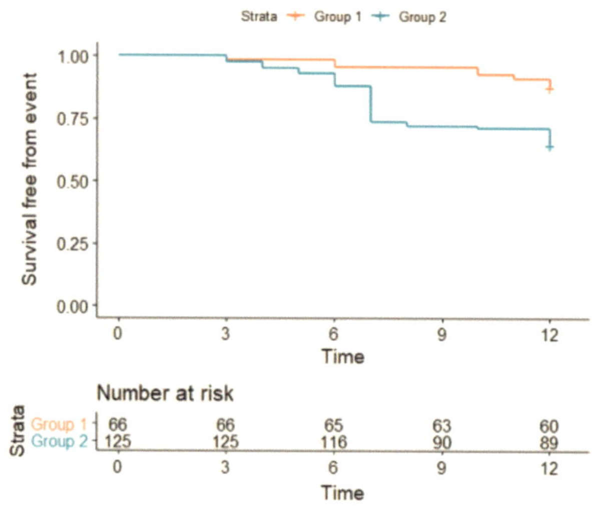

Figure 9.
K-M curve showing survival free from AT/AF recurrence with or without AAD in both groups. From Lai et al. [32].

mitral isthmus and improves long-term results if systematically added to conventional strategies in setting of persistent atrial fibrillation ablation. Results of randomized clinical trials adding VOM-ETHO to pulmonary vein ablation (VENUS AF) and PVI plus linear lesions (Marshall-PLAN) demonstrates beneficial impact of long-term sinus rhythm maintenance in patients with persistent atrial fibrillation.

Author details

Andrea Rossi[1]*, Procolo Marchese[2] and Marcello Piacenti[1]

1 Electrophysiology Unit, "Fondazione Toscana Gabriele Monasterio", Pisa, Italy

2 Electrophysiology Department, "G.C. Mazzoni" Hospital, Ascoli Piceno, Italy

*Address all correspondence to: andrea.rossi@ftgm.it

References

[1] Lee SH, Tai CT, Hsieh MH, et al. Predictors of non-pulmonary vein ectopic beats initiating paroxysmal atrial fibrillation. Journal of the American College of Cardiology. 2005;**46**(6):1054-1059

[2] Vlachos K, Denis A, Takigawa M, et al. The role of Marshall bundle epicardial connections in atrial tachycardias after atrial fibrillation ablation. Heart Rhythm. 2019;**16**(9):1341-1347

[3] Ulphani JS, Arora R, Cain JH, et al. The ligament of Marshall as a parasympathetic conduit. American Journal of Physiology. Heart and Circulatory Physiology. 2007;**293**:1629-1635

[4] Baez-Escudero J, Takehiko K, Amish D. Ethanol infusion in the vein of Marshall leads to parasympathetic denervation of the human left Atrium. Journal of the American College of Cardiology. 2014;**63**(18):1892-1901

[5] Kim DT, Lai AC, Hwang C, et al. The ligament of Marshall: A structural analysis in human hearts with implications for atrial arrhythmias. Journal of the American College of Cardiology. 2000;**36**:1324-1327

[6] Kamanu S, Tan AY, Peter CT, et al. Vein of Marshall activity during sustained atrial fibrillation. Journal of Cardiovascular Electrophysiology. 2006;**17**:839-846

[7] Nakashima T, Pambrun T, Vlachos K, et al. Impact of vein of Marshall ethanol infusion on mitral isthmus block efficacy and durability. Circulation Arrhythmia and Electrophysiology. 2020;**13e008884**:1435-1442

[8] Marshall J. On the development of the great anterior veins in man and mammalia: including an account of certain remnants of foetal structure found in the adult, a comparative view of these great veins in the different mammalia, and an analysis of their occasional peculiarities in the human subject. Philosophical Transactions. Royal Society of London. 1850;**140**:133-169

[9] Valderrabano M, Morales PF, Rodriguez-Manero M, et al. The human left atrial venous circulation as a vascular route for atrial pharmacological therapies. Effect of ethanol infusion. Journal of the American College of Cardiology. 2017;**3**(9):1-13

[10] Kamakura T, Derval N, Duchateau J, et al. Vein of Marshall ethanol infusion. Feasibility, pitfalls, and complications in over 700 patients. Circulation Arrhythmia and Electrophysiology. 2021;**14**:719-728

[11] Valderrabano M, Chen HR, Sidhu J, et al. Retrograde ethanol infusion in the vein of Marshall. Regional left atrial ablation, vagal denervation and feasibility in humans. Circulation. Arrhythmia and Electrophysiology. 2009;**2**:50-56

[12] Báez-Escudero JL, Keida T, Dave AS, Okishige K, Valderrábano M. Ethanol infusion in the vein of Marshall leads to parasympathetic denervation of the human left atrium. Journal of the American College of Cardiology. 2014;**63**(18):1892-1901

[13] Báez-Escudero JL, Morales PF, Dave AS, et al. Ethanol infusion in the vein of Marshall facilitates mitral isthmus ablation. Heart Rhythm Journal. 2012;**9**(8):1207-1215

[14] Chugh A, Gurm HS, Krishnasamy K, et al. Spectrum of atrial arrhythmias

using the ligament of Marshall in patients with atrial fibrillation. Heart Rhythm Journal. 2018;**15**(1):17-24

[15] Hwang C, Wu TJ, Doshi RN, et al. Vein of marshall cannulation for the analysis of electrical activity in patients with focal atrial fibrillation. Circulation. 2000;**101**(13):1503-1505

[16] Valderrábano M, Morales PF, Rodríguez-Mañero M, et al. The human left atrial venous circulation as a vascular route for atrial pharmacological therapies. JACC Clinical Electrophysiology. 2017;**3**(9):1020-1032

[17] Kitamura T, Vlachos K, Denis A, et al. Ethanol infusion forMarshall bundle epicardial connections in Marshall bundle-related atrial tachycardias following atrial fibrillation ablation: The accessibility and success rate of ethanol infusion by using a femoral approach. Journal of Cardiovascular Electrophysiology. 2019;**9**:1-9

[18] Valderrábano M, Peterson LE, Swarup V, et al. Effect of Catheter Ablation With Vein of Marshall Ethanol Infusion vs Catheter Ablation Alone on Persistent Atrial Fibrillation The VENUS Randomized Clinical Trial. Journal of the American Medical Association. 2020;**324**(16):1620-1628

[19] Chugh A, Oral H, Lemola K, et al. Prevalence, mechanisms, and clinical significance of macroreentrant atrial tachycardia during and following left atrial ablation for atrial fibrillation. Heart Rhythm. 2005;**2**:464-471

[20] Yokokawa M, Latchamsetty R, Ghanbari H, et al. Characteristics of atrial tachycardia due to small vs large reentrant circuits after ablation of persistent atrial fibrillation. Heart Rhythm. 2013;**10**:469-476

[21] Takigawa M, Derval N, Maury P, et al. Comprehensive multicenter study of the common isthmus in post-atrial fibrillation ablation multiple-loop atrial tachy-cardia. Circulation. Arrhythmia and Electrophysiology. 2018;**11**:1-15

[22] Han S, Joung B, Scanavacca M, et al. Electrophysiological characteristics of the Marshall bundle in humans. Heart Rhythm. 2010;7:786-793

[23] Vlachos K, Denis A, Takigawa M, et al. The role of Marshall bundle epicardial connection in atrial tachycardias after atrial fibrillation ablation. Heart Rhythm. 2019;**16**(9):1341-1347

[24] Scherlag BJ, Yeh BK, Robinson MJ. Inferior interatrial pathway in the dog. Circulation Research. 1972;**31**:18-35

[25] Lee JH, Nam GB, Kim M, et al. Radiofrequency catheter ablation targeting the vein of Marshall in difficult mitral isthmus ablation or pulmonary vein isolation. Journal of Cardiovascular Electrophysiology. 2017;**28**:386-393

[26] Baez-Escudero JL, Morales PF, Dave AS, et al. Ethanol infusion in the vein of Marshall facilitates mitral isthmus ablation. Heart Rhythm. 2012;**9**:1207-1215

[27] Valderrabano M, Liu X, Sasaridis C, et al. Ethanol infusion in the vein of Marshall: Adjunctive effects during ablation of atrial fibrillation. Heart Rhythm. 2009;**6**:1552-1558

[28] Thompson N, Kitamura T, Martin R, et al. Demonstration of persistent conduction across the mitral isthmus via the vein of Marshall with high- density activation mapping. Circulation. Arrhythmia and Electrophysiology. 2017;**10**:e005152

[29] Lador A, Peterson LE, Swarup V, et al. Determinants of outcome impact of vein of Marshall ethanol infusion when added to catheter ablation of persistent atrial fibrillation: a secondary analysis of the VENUS randomized clinical trial. Heart Rhythm. 2021;**19**:S1547-S5271

[30] Derval N, Duchateau J, Denis A, et al. Marshall bundle elimination, Pulmonary vein isolation, and Line completion for anatomical ablation of persistent atrial fibrillation (Marshall-PLAN): prospective, single-center study. Heart Rhythm. 2021;**18**(4):529-537

[31] Liu XX, Sang CH, Long DY, et al. Prospective randomized comparison between upgraded '2C3L' vs. PVI approach for catheter ablation of persistent atrial fibrillation: PROMPT-AF trial design. Pacing and Clinical Electrophysiology. 2021;**44**(9):1651

[32] Lai Y, Liu XX, Sang CH, et al. Effectiveness of ethanol infusion into the vein of Marshall combined with a fixed anatomical ablation strategy (the "upgraded 2C3L" approach) for catheter ablation of persistent atrial fibrillation. Journal of Cardiovascular Electrophysiology. 2021;**32**(7):1849-1856

Chapter 10

Concomitant Atrial Fibrillation Surgery

Chawannuch Ruaengsri and Suchart Chaiyaroj

Abstract

Atrial fibrillation (AF) is the most common cardiac arrhythmia and is the major cause of stroke and heart failure. The treatment options of AF include medical treatment and catheter-based or surgical ablation. Cox et al. introduced the Cox-Maze procedure (the cut-and-sew Maze) that was first performed clinically in 1987 at Barnes Jewish Hospital, St. Louis, MO. This procedure is characterized by multiple incisions created at both left and right atria to terminate AF while allowing the electrical impulse generated from sino-atrial node to atrioventricular node. The Cox-Maze IV is the latest iteration developed by Damiano Jr. et al., which replaced the previous cut-and-sew Maze with a combination of less invasive linear lesions achieved by new ablation technology, the bipolar radiofrequency (RF), and cryoablation. This chapter describes the operative techniques, preoperative planning, indication for surgery, and future option of surgical treatment.

Keywords: atrial fibrillation, Cox-Maze, surgical ablation, cardiac surgery

1. Introduction

Atrial fibrillation (AF) is the most common cardiac arrhythmia and is the major cause of stroke. Over the past several decades, AF surgical Ablation has become a treatment option for refractory and debilitating cardiac arrhythmias. Surgical innovation and ablation technology has rapidly evolved and has revolutionized therapies for AF. Although indications for surgical ablation have narrowed, AF surgery remains an important and effective treatment option.

Medical treatment has had many shortcomings including both the inefficacy and unwanted side effects of many antiarrhythmic drugs [1]. Initial attempts aimed at providing rate control failed the development of catheter and surgical ablation in the 1980s. After a decade of experimental studies, the Maze procedure was introduced in 1987. It has gone through several modifications and has become the gold standard for the treatment of AF [2].

2. Previous surgical ablation

2.1 The left atrial isolation procedure

In 1980, Dr. James Cox developed the left atrial isolation at Duke University. This is the first surgical procedure designed specifically to eliminate AF. This procedure confined AF to the left atrium, allowing the remainder of the heart to be in sinus rhythm [3–5].

2.2 The Corridor procedure

In 1985, Guiraudon et al. developed the corridor procedure to isolate a strip of atrial septum including both the sinoatrial and atrioventricular nodes to allow the sinoatrial node to pace both right and left ventricles [6]. The shortcomings of the corridor procedure included failure to prevent thromboembolism as well as atrio-ventricular dyssynchrony. It did have the advantage of preserving atrioventricular conduction [6].

2.3 The atrial transection procedure

Cox et al. first described the atrial transection procedure in 1985. Using a canine model, they found that a single longitudinal incision around both atria and down into the septum would terminate AF [4, 7]. This procedure effectively prevents AF or atrial flutter in animals but not in humans. Although this procedure was abandoned, it represented a transitional step toward the Cox-Maze procedure.

2.4 The Cox-Maze procedure

After extensive animal studies, The Cox-Maze procedure was introduced clinically by James Cox in 1987 [2, 4]. This procedure was designed based on the theory that macro-reentrant circuits cause and propagate AF. The Cox-Maze procedure restored sinus rhythm as well as AV synchrony, reducing the risk of stroke and thromboembolism [8]. The original of Cox-Maze procedure, The Cox-Maze I, consisted of multiple surgical incisions across both atria that allowed for a pathway for the sinus impulse to reach the AV node. It permitted depolarization of most of the atrial myocardium resulting in preservation of most of the atrial contractile function [9].

The Cox-Maze II was formulated because the Cox-Maze I had problems with late chronotropic incompetence with a high incidence of pacemaker implantation [10].

The Cox-Maze III proved to be effective and became the gold standard for surgical treatment of AF [1, 2]. The procedure is often called the cut-and-sew maze, and the surgical results of the Cox-Maze III were excellent, with over 90% of patients free from symptomatic AF at late follow up [11–14]. Despite its efficacy, the cut-and-sew maze was technically difficult and required a lengthy period of aortic cross clamp time, which limited its widespread adoption. Over the last two decades, modern ablation devices transformed the Cox-Maze III into an easier, shorter, and less invasive procedure, which has been termed the Cox-Maze IV. These have allowed for more widespread adoption [15]. These modern technologies have been used to replace the surgical incisions and have allowed the development of less invasive approaches.

3. Surgical ablation technology

When ablation technology was introduced, the goal was to replace the incision lines of the Cox-Maze III as much as possible. An ablation technology had to have

3 characteristics in order to replicate a surgical incision. First, a device had to create a line of bidirectional conduction block. A pattern of lesions with these properties can prevent AF, either through blocking macro or micro-reentrant circuits or by isolating focal triggers. Only transmural lesions produce reliable conduction block, as even small gaps in ablation lines retain the ability to conduct both sinus and fibrillatory impulses [16, 17]. Second, the ablation device had to be safe. Safety requires that the device delivers a precise dose of energy to minimize both inadequate ablation and potential injury to nearby vital structures by excessive ablation. Lastly, the ablation device had to make AF surgery simpler and require less operative time compared to the original technique.

Several ablation technologies have been developed, and each has its relative advantages and disadvantages. Cryoablation and bipolar radiofrequency (RF) devices have been shown to be the most effective and are the ablation technologies used for the Cox-Maze IV [18].

3.1 Cryoablation

Cryoablation technology creates ablation lines by freezing myocardial issue. Cryoablation preserves the myocardial fibrous skeleton and collagen structure, making it one of the safest energy sources available. These devices work by pumping a liquid refrigerant to the tip of a device where it undergoes evaporation, and in the process absorbing heat from the tissue in contact with the tip. This causes intracellular and extracellular water to freeze. The resulting ice crystals disrupt the plasma membrane and cause early cell death via cell lysis. Lesions also expand due to induced apoptosis. The size of the lesion produced depends on the thermal conductivity and temperature of both the probe and the tissue [19].

Two commercially available sources of cryothermal energy are in clinical use in cardiac surgery. Nitrous oxide-based devices are manufactured by AtriCure (Cincinnati, OH). Devices using Argon have been developed and are currently distributed by Medtronic (Minneapolis, MN). The minimum temperature that can be produced by an ablation device is limited by the thermodynamic properties of the refrigerant used. At 1 atmosphere of pressure, nitrous oxide is capable of cooling tissue to −89.5°C, whereas argon can cool tissue to −185.7°C. Nitrous oxide based cryoablation has a long history of clinical use with a well-defined efficacy and is safe except around the coronary arteries [20, 21]. Experimental and clinical studies have shown intimal hyperplasia and coronary artery stenosis after cryoablation [21–23]. The disadvantage of cryoablation is the relatively longer time required to create transmural lesion (usually 2–3 minutes). There is also difficulty in creating lesions on beating heart from an epicardial approach due to the circulating blood acts as a heat sink effect [24]. Moreover, freezing of intra-atrial blood poses a potential risk of thromboembolism.

The nitrous oxide technology can be used with both the rigid, reusable, and the flexible, disposable probes. The argon technology is available only as a flexible, disposable ablation device.

3.2 Radiofrequency energy

Radiofrequency (RF) has been used for many years by cardiac electrophysiologists and surgeons to ablate cardiac tissue. RF energy can be delivered using unipolar or bipolar electrodes.

3.3 Unipolar RF

Energy is delivered between the tip of electrode and a grounding pad attached to the patient. Unlike bipolar RF energy, an alternating amount is delivered between 2 jaws of a clamp. Several factors contributed to lesion size such as tissue contact area, interface temperature, the amount of power applied and duration of energy delivery. Several factors can limit the depth of the lesion, potentially preventing successful creation of a transmural lesion with conduction block. These include char formation, epicardial fat, myocardial and endovascular blood flow, and tissue thickness. Several unipolar RF ablation devices have been developed. These include dry, irrigated and suction assisted devices. These devices have had limited applicability in cardiac surgery. Transmural lesions can be created with dry unipolar RF on the arrested heart in animal studies. Unfortunately, this has not been reproducible in clinical practices [25]. There is one study that confirmed that only 20% of transmural lesions achieved after 2 minutes of ablation time during mitral valve surgery. Moreover, the results of epicardial unipolar RF ablation on the beating heart were found to be even less successful. Another animal study has demonstrated the epicardial unipolar RF failed to create transmural lesions on the beating heart [26]. One clinical study has shown only 10% success rate of transmural lesions achieved after epicardial RF ablation [27]. Convection caused by circulating blood that explained the failure of epicardial unipolar RF ablation on the beating heart [28, 29]. No unipolar RF device has been shown by independent laboratories to be capable of reliably creating transmural lesions on the beating heart [30]. The recent expert consensus guidelines mentioned that the use of epicardial unipolar RF ablation outside of clinical trials is not recommended because its efficacy remains questionable [31].

3.4 Bipolar RF

The electrodes are embedded in the jaws of a clamp to focus the delivery of energy. Multiple studies have shown bipolar RF ablation to be able to create transmural lesions on the beating heart in animals and humans with short ablation times [32–34]. Bipolar RF devices are currently sold by two companies in United States (AtriCure, West Chester, OH and Medtronic, Minneapolis, MN). Both devices have shown similar experimental and clinical efficacy. Bipolar RF energy also has a more favorable safety profile compared to unipolar RF. Some clinical complications of unipolar RF devices have been reported including coronary vessel injuries, stroke and esophageal perforation leading to atrioesophageal fistula [35–39]. There have been no collateral injuries reported after bipolar RF technology despite its widespread clinical use. Innovation continues within the field of RF ablation technology, including the development of unipolar-bipolar hybrid devices. The Cobra Fusion (AtriCure, West Chester, OH) a suction-assisted device that combines bipolar and unipolar RF, has been shown in early experimental reports to have improved efficacy in creating transmural epicardial lesions on the beating heart [40].

The recent expert consensus guidelines state that the best evidence exists for the use of bipolar radiofrequency (RF) clamps and cryoablation devices, which have become integral parts of many procedures, including pulmonary vein isolation and the Cox-Maze IV procedure.

Bipolar RF clamps or cryoprobes (both reusable and/or disposable) are recommended to be used for PVI in both empty arrested and beating heart with exit block confirmation testing. For beating heart, endocardial cryoablation is recommended for free wall linear ablation instead of epicardial cryoablation due to higher success rate of transmurality. The guidelines also suggest to identify and avoid injury to coronary vessels while doing ablation with any devices [31].

Other energy delivery devices including microwave, laser, and ultrasound have been used clinically but limitations of these technologies have led to limited use and withdrawal of these devices from the market [28, 41–45].

4. Indication for surgical atrial fibrillation ablation

A recent consensus statement described current indications for surgical ablation of AF include

1. All symptomatic AF patients undergoing concomitant cardiac surgery

2. Selected asymptomatic AF patients undergoing concomitant cardiac surgery which the ablation can be performed by experienced surgeons; and

3. Symptomatic AF patients who have failed medical treatment or have recurrent AF after catheter ablation and prefer stand-alone surgical approach [46].

Strong evidence showing an association between AF and increased mortality and morbidity has led to recent expert consensus guidelines to recommend surgical ablation at the time of concomitant cardiac procedures to restore sinus rhythm with a Class I or IIa indication [31, 47]. Addition of concomitant surgical ablation for AF does improve health-related quality of life (HRQL) and AF-related symptom. It also improves short-term and long-term survival [31].

Some relative indications for surgery that were mentioned in AF surgery expert institutions are persistent AF patients with high risk for stroke and CHADS2 score ≥ 2 and inability to take life-long and anticoagulation and persistent AF patients with proper anticoagulation but still have had a cerebrovascular event [2].

Recent consensus guidelines recommend addition of a concomitant surgical ablation procedure for AF does not change the incidence of perioperative or late stroke/TIA (class IIa) but subgroup analysis of nonrandomized controlled trials found a significant reduction in late stroke/TIA incidence [31].

5. Surgical technique

There are several procedures that are currently performed to treat AF: the Cox-Maze IV procedure, left atrial lesion sets, pulmonary vein isolation (PVI), and hybrid ablations.

5.1 The Cox-Maze IV procedure

The Cox-Maze IV replicates the Cut-and-sew Maze lesion set using bipolar RF energy and cryoablation to replace most of the incisions in the Cox-Maze III [2, 48]. Clinical results have shown that the Cox-Maze IV achieves the high success rate of the Cox-Maze III with significant reduction in operative time and lower complication rates [2, 49]. The Cox-Maze IV procedure requires cardiopulmonary bypass. It can be performed either through a median sternotomy or a minimally invasive right thoracotomy approach. The selection of an approach should be based on the presence of concomitant cardiac pathology, patient-specific anatomic characteristics and the experience of the surgeon [2]. Patients who are in AF at the time of surgery and have no intracardiac thrombosis on intraoperative transesophageal echocardiogram are electrically cardioverted and started on intravenous amiodarone. Pacing thresholds are measured from each pulmonary vein [2, 50].

5.2 Median sternotomy approach

For the standard fashion, the right and left pulmonary veins are bluntly dissected, mobilized and encircled with umbilical tapes. Amiodarone is given and electrical cardioversion is performed if the patient is in AF. Pacing thresholds are performed and pulmonary veins isolation (PVI) is achieved using bipolar clamps. After PVI is completed, exit block is confirmed from each pulmonary vein [2, 50].

To perform the right atrial lesion set, the patient is then cooled to 34°C. Lesions from right atrial lesion set are performed on the beating heart. Two purse-string sutures are created at the base of both right and left atrial appendage which is large enough to place a jaw of bipolar RF clamp. Right atrial free wall ablation is first performed through the previously made purse-string suture down toward the aortic side of the right atrial appendage. Right atriotomy is created vertically toward the atrioventricular (AV) groove. Superior and Inferior vena cava lesions are performed using RF clamp applying from inferior aspect of previous right atriotomy incision. Next, endocardial ablation is created using a linear cryoprobe starting from the right atriotomy down onto the 2 o'clock position of the tricuspid annulus. Then another endocardial ablation lesion is performed using the linear cryoprobe inserted through the previous made purse-string suture down to the 10 o'clock position of tricuspid annulus (this lesion can be omitted in case of small right atrium and no tricuspid regurgitation) [2, 50].

After the aortic clamp is on and the heart is completely arrested, the left atrial lesions set is performed. The left atrial appendage is identified and amputated, and an ablation is performed through the amputated left atrial appendage. The bipolar RF clamp is used to create a connecting lesion into the left inferior or superior pulmonary vein. The left atrial appendage is then oversewn in a double layer. Methylene blue is then used to mark the coronary sinus. Then left atriotomy incision is made, the roof and floor lesions are created with bipolar RF clamp. From the inferior margin of left atriotomy, bipolar RF clamp is applied to create ablation line toward the mitral annulus and across the coronary sinus. A bell-shaped cryoprobe is used to make and endocardial lesion to the mitral annulus at the end of the mitral isthmus lesion. An epicardial cryoablation is performed over the coronary sinus in line with the endocardial lesion to complete the left atrial isthmus lesion [2]. Some institutes use only cryoablation to create the Cox-Maze IV lesion set. The atriotomy is then closed. The patient is weaned from cardiopulmonary bypass and the sternotomy closed in a standard fashion.

5.3 Right minithoracotomy approach

The patient is intubated with a double-lumen endotracheal tube with right lung deflation. Femoral cannulation is obtained for cardiopulmonary bypass. A small minithoracotomy is performed over the fourth intercostal space, midaxillary line. For the right minithoracotomy approach, the ablation lesions set remains the same. The right atrial lesion ablation is performed through 3 purse-string sutures as in a minimally invasive approach. In case of left atrial lesion set, the pattern of ablation also remains the same except for the left pulmonary vein isolation is performed endocardially using cryoablation probe to connect the superior and inferior box lesions. The left atrial appendage exclusion is performed by double layer oversewing endocardially.

5.4 Cox-Maze IV surgical result

The Cox-Maze III procedure had excellent success rates for the treatment of AF. One of the studies at Washington University examined the outcomes of 198 patients who underwent the Cox-Maze III procedure. Their study showed a 97% freedom from symptomatic AF with a mean follow up of 5.4 years and no difference in recurrence when comparing patients who received a stand-alone Cox-Maze III versus patients who received a concomitant procedure [32]. Similar results have been obtained from other studies with the cut-and-sew method [12, 14, 51]. However, very few of these patients had prolonged monitoring or even follow-up electrocardiograms or prolonged monitoring to assess the rhythm.

The modification of the Cox-Maze IV simplified the traditional procedure and made it easier to perform. This allowed for the development of minimally invasive approaches and more widespread adoption, allowing for many more patients to receive surgical ablation at the time of concomitant surgery [52]. In 2018, the number of patients had increased to more than 30,000 by estimates using the Society of Thoracic Surgeons (STS) Adult cardiac surgery database [47, 52]. Badhwar et al reported an overall increase of 50% in performing concomitant surgical ablation from the year of 2011–2014 [47, 52].

The recent study from Damiano group demonstrated an excellent long-term efficacy at maintaining sinus rhythm of the Cox-Maze IV with 77% overall freedom from recurrent ATAs at 10 years follow-up [52]. Moreover, at late follow-up, the results of the Cox-Maze IV remained superior to those reported for catheter ablation and other forms of surgical ablation for AF [52].

The findings from other studies also support the recommendation that the Cox-Maze IV should be considered in all patients undergoing concomitant cardiac surgery if it can be performed without adding morbidity or mortality to the procedure [52–56].

5.5 Left atrial procedures

Most centers have advocated performing ablation confined to the atrium only to treat AF. Since the majority of paroxysmal AF appears to originate from the pulmonary veins and the posterior of left atrium. Left atrial lesion set typically involves pulmonary vein isolation, with a lesion to the mitral annulus and the left atrial appendage removal/exclusion. The advantage of avoiding right atrial lesions is a potential of lower rate of postoperative pacemaker implantation [57]. However, Gillinov et al. published a large series demonstrating the omission of the left atrial isthmus lesion resulted in a significantly higher incidence of recurrent AF in persistent AF patients [58]. To complete this isthmus lesion, it is important to ablate the coronary sinus in line with the endocardial lesion. Some studies have shown that isolation of the entire posterior left atrium is associated with improved outcomes compared with isolation of the pulmonary veins alone and had significantly higher rate freedom from AF when compared with left atrial set alone [59, 60]. Some studies have shown that AF can originate from the right atrium in up to 30% [61–63].

5.6 Pulmonary vein isolation (PVI)

Pulmonary vein isolation can be performed without cardiopulmonary bypass with minimally invasive technique via either minithoracotomy or thoracoscopy and can be easily added to other cardiac surgical procedure. Haissaguerre study documented that the triggers for paroxysmal AF originate from pulmonary veins in the majority of cases [64]. However, up to 30% of triggers may originate outside the pulmonary veins [65]. This is further informed by anatomic substrates that could be the generation of AF as extrapulmonary triggers located at the superior vena cava, the ligament of Marshall, and the epicardial ridge between the left pulmonary vein and the left atrial appendage [66]. The pulmonary veins can be isolated separately or as a box lesion. The most common approach for treatment of lone AF uses an endoscopic, port-based approach. Bipolar RF clamps are favored but unipolar RF, cryoablation, and high-intensity focused ultrasound devices have also been used [43, 67, 68]. Although energy sources such as microwave proved not to deliver effective lesions [69]. The application of RF bipolar clamp to create PVI antral pairs via bilateral thoracotomies has been established as a safe procedure with reasonable short-term efficacy [70]. There is a study that demonstrated the late gaps in ablation lines occurred after epicardial PVI ablation regardless of previously exit block confirming intraoperatively [17]. This could be a supporting idea of beneficial combining epicardial PVI with endocardial ablation [31]. The FAST trial, a multicenter randomized trial, compared 63 patients who received linear antral pulmonary vein isolation by catheter ablation and 61 patients who received bipolar RF PVI and ganglion plexus ablation. Most patients had paroxysmal AF. At 1 year, freedom from left atrial arrhythmia without ATA was 66% for surgical ablation versus 36% for catheter ablation [71].

This procedure will be completed until the left atrial appendage has been addressed. In the past, this had been done by stapling across the base of the left atrial appendage. This requires careful surgical technique and attention due to it can result in tears and bleeding [72]. Clip devices have been developed to address this difficulty. They improved efficacy and safety when compared to staplers [73, 74].

5.7 Hybrid ablations

To lessen the invasiveness of surgical ablation, extended epicardial ablation was introduced, which can be placed through thoracoscopic ports. However, these probes have not been able to achieve the same degree of transmurality created by bipolar clamps [30]. This led to the idea of combining endocardial ablation via transcatheter techniques and epicardial ablation via surgical techniques in a hybrid approach. Based on current experience, the hybrid approach with the most effective outcomes and safety profile appears to be bilateral pulmonary vein procedures performed surgically with left atrial appendage management combined with different endocardial ablation protocol [31]. The principles of these approaches are based on the understanding that it is possible to apply mapping techniques from electrophysiologists to surgical epicardial ablation techniques when performed on beating heart [31].

Currently, there are several procedures being performed surgically, combining with endocardial ablation e.g., PVI procedures either bilateral thoracoscopic/minithoracotomy approach or unilateral thoracoscopic PVI posterior encircling box lesion with or without left atrial appendage management. There is also an alternative approach to posterior left atrial wall epicardial ablation lesion (pericardioscopic epicardial debulking ablation procedures, also known as "convergent method") [31].

The recent expert guideline favors the hybrid approach over percutaneous catheter ablation in terms of results in a subgroup of symptomatic AF patients who have had failed medical and percutaneous catheter ablation treatment [31].

6. Conclusion

The ideal surgical procedure for AF would be a minimally invasive procedure that does not require cardiopulmonary bypass and should preserve normal atrial physiology, have minimal morbidity, and have a high success rate. Achieving this goal will require a better understanding of the mechanism of AF in individual patients and tailoring of treatment approaches. This would have significant advantages and prevent both over and under-ablation. This will require better preoperative diagnostics to identify mechanisms of AF. Non-invasive ECG imaging has a great potential in this era [75, 76] that could be beneficial to tailor lesion sets as well as to decide which specific ablation modalities for individual patients.

Author details

Chawannuch Ruaengsri[1] and Suchart Chaiyaroj[2]*

1 Stanford University, Stanford, CA, USA

2 Faculty of Medicine, Department of Surgery, Ramathibodi Hospital, Mahidol University, Bangkok, Thailand

*Address all correspondence to: schaiyaroj@gmail.com

References

[1] Calkins H, Hindricks G, Cappato R, Kim YH, Saad EB, Aguinaga L, et al. 2017 HRS/EHRA/ECAS/APHRS/SOLAECE expert consensus statement on catheter and surgical ablation of atrial fibrillation: Executive summary. Journal of Arrhythmia. 2017;**33**(5):369-409

[2] Ruaengsri C, Schill MR, Khiabani AJ, Schuessler RB, Melby SJ, Damiano RJ. The Cox-maze IV procedure in its second decade: Still the gold standard? European Journal of Cardiothoracic Surgery. 2018;**53**(1):i19-i25

[3] Williams JM, Ungerleider RM, Lofland GK, Cox JL. Left atrial isolation: New technique for the treatment of supraventricular arrhythmias. The Journal of Thoracic and Cardiovascular Surgery. 1980;**80**(3):373-380

[4] Cox JL. The surgical treatment of atrial fibrillation. IV. Surgical technique. The Journal of Thoracic and Cardiovascular Surgery. 1991;**101**(4):584-592

[5] Cox JL, Canavan TE, Schuessler RB, Cain ME, Lindsay BD, Stone C, et al. The surgical treatment of atrial fibrillation. II. Intraoperative electrophysiologic mapping and description of the electrophysiologic basis of atrial flutter and atrial fibrillation. The Journal of Thoracic and Cardiovascular Surgery. 1991;**101**(3):406-426

[6] Defauw JJ, Guiraudon GM, van Hemel NM, Vermeulen FE, Kingma JH, de Bakker JM. Surgical therapy of paroxysmal atrial fibrillation with the "corridor" operation. The Annals of Thoracic Surgery. 1992;**53**(4):564-570

[7] Smith PK, Holman WL, Cox JL. Surgical treatment of supraventricular tachyarrhythmias. The Surgical Clinics of North America. 1985;**65**(3):553-570

[8] Cox JL, Ad N, Palazzo T. Impact of the maze procedure on the stroke rate in patients with atrial fibrillation. The Journal of Thoracic and Cardiovascular Surgery. 1999;**118**(5):833-840

[9] Feinberg MS, Waggoner AD, Kater KM, Cox JL, Lindsay BD, Perez JE. Restoration of atrial function after the maze procedure for patients with atrial fibrillation. Assessment by Doppler echocardiography. Circulation. 1994;**90**(5 Pt 2):II285-II292

[10] Edgerton ZJ, Edgerton JR. History of surgery for atrial fibrillation. Heart Rhythm. 2009;**6**(12 Suppl):S1-S4

[11] Prasad SM, Maniar HS, Camillo CJ, Schuessler RB, Boineau JP, Sundt TM 3rd, et al. The Cox maze III procedure for atrial fibrillation: Long-term efficacy in patients undergoing lone versus concomitant procedures. The Journal of Thoracic and Cardiovascular Surgery. 2003;**126**(6):1822-1828

[12] McCarthy PM, Gillinov AM, Castle L, Chung M, Cosgrove D 3rd. The Cox-Maze procedure: The Cleveland Clinic experience. Seminars in Thoracic and Cardiovascular Surgery. 2000;**12**(1):25-29

[13] Raanani E, Albage A, David TE, Yau TM, Armstrong S. The efficacy of the Cox/maze procedure combined with mitral valve surgery: A matched control study. European Journal of Cardio-Thoracic Surgery. 2001;**19**(4):438-442

[14] Schaff HV, Dearani JA, Daly RC, Orszulak TA, Danielson GK. Cox-Maze procedure for atrial fibrillation:

Mayo Clinic experience. Seminars in Thoracic and Cardiovascular Surgery. 2000;**12**(1):30-37

[15] Gammie JS, Haddad M, Milford-Beland S, Welke KF, Ferguson TB Jr, O'Brien SM, et al. Atrial fibrillation correction surgery: Lessons from the Society of Thoracic Surgeons National Cardiac Database. The Annals of Thoracic Surgery. 2008;**85**(3):909-914

[16] Ishii Y, Nitta T, Sakamoto S, Tanaka S, Asano G. Incisional atrial reentrant tachycardia: Experimental study on the conduction property through the isthmus. The Journal of Thoracic and Cardiovascular Surgery. 2003;**126**(1):254-262

[17] Melby SJ, Lee AM, Zierer A, Kaiser SP, Livhits MJ, Boineau JP, et al. Atrial fibrillation propagates through gaps in ablation lines: Implications for ablative treatment of atrial fibrillation. Heart Rhythm. 2008;**5**(9):1296-1301

[18] Robertson JO, Lawrance CP, Maniar HS, Damiano RJ Jr. Surgical techniques used for the treatment of atrial fibrillation. Circulation Journal. 2013;**77**(8):1941-1951

[19] Melby SJ, Schuessler RB, Damiano RJ Jr. Ablation technology for the surgical treatment of atrial fibrillation. ASAIO Journal. 2013;**59**(5):461-468

[20] Gage AM, Montes M, Gage AA. Freezing the canine thoracic aorta in situ. The Journal of Surgical Research. 1979;**27**(5):331-340

[21] Holman WL, Ikeshita M, Ungerleider RM, Smith PK, Ideker RE, Cox JL. Cryosurgery for cardiac arrhythmias: Acute and chronic effects on coronary arteries. The American Journal of Cardiology. 1983;**51**(1):149-155

[22] Watanabe H, Hayashi J, Aizawa Y. Myocardial infarction after cryoablation surgery for Wolff-Parkinson-White syndrome. The Japanese Journal of Thoracic and Cardiovascular Surgery. 2002;**50**(5):210-212

[23] Manasse E, Colombo P, Roncalli M, Gallotti R. Myocardial acute and chronic histological modifications induced by cryoablation. European Journal of Cardio-Thoracic Surgery. 2000;**17**(3):339-340

[24] Aupperle H, Doll N, Walther T, Kornherr P, Ullmann C, Schoon HA, et al. Ablation of atrial fibrillation and esophageal injury: Effects of energy source and ablation technique. The Journal of Thoracic and Cardiovascular Surgery. 2005;**130**(6):1549-1554

[25] Santiago T, Melo JQ, Gouveia RH, Martins AP. Intra-atrial temperatures in radiofrequency endocardial ablation: Histologic evaluation of lesions. The Annals of Thoracic Surgery. 2003;**75**(5):1495-1501

[26] Thomas SP, Guy DJ, Boyd AC, Eipper VE, Ross DL, Chard RB. Comparison of epicardial and endocardial linear ablation using handheld probes. The Annals of Thoracic Surgery. 2003;**75**(2):543-548

[27] Santiago T, Melo J, Gouveia RH, Neves J, Abecasis M, Adragao P, et al. Epicardial radiofrequency applications: In vitro and in vivo studies on human atrial myocardium. European Journal of Cardio-Thoracic Surgery. 2003;**24**(4):481-486

[28] Melby SJ, Zierer A, Kaiser SP, Schuessler RB, Damiano RJ Jr. Epicardial microwave ablation on the beating heart for atrial fibrillation: The dependency of lesion depth on cardiac output. The Journal of Thoracic and Cardiovascular Surgery. 2006;**132**(2):355-360

[29] Gaynor SL, Byrd GD, Diodato MD, Ishii Y, Lee AM, Prasad SM, et al. Microwave ablation for atrial fibrillation: Dose-response curves in the cardioplegia-arrested and beating heart. The Annals of Thoracic Surgery. 2006;**81**(1):72-76

[30] Schuessler RB, Lee AM, Melby SJ, Voeller RK, Gaynor SL, Sakamoto S, et al. Animal studies of epicardial atrial ablation. Heart Rhythm. 2009;**6**(12 Suppl):S41-S45

[31] Ad N, Damiano RJ Jr, Badhwar V, Calkins H, La Meir M, Nitta T, et al. Expert consensus guidelines: Examining surgical ablation for atrial fibrillation. The Journal of Thoracic and Cardiovascular Surgery. 2017;**153**(6):1330-1354

[32] Gaynor SL, Diodato MD, Prasad SM, Ishii Y, Schuessler RB, Bailey MS, et al. A prospective, single-center clinical trial of a modified Cox maze procedure with bipolar radiofrequency ablation. The Journal of Thoracic and Cardiovascular Surgery. 2004;**128**(4):535-542

[33] Prasad SM, Maniar HS, Diodato MD, Schuessler RB, Damiano RJ Jr. Physiological consequences of bipolar radiofrequency energy on the atria and pulmonary veins: A chronic animal study. The Annals of Thoracic Surgery. 2003;**76**(3):836-841

[34] Prasad SM, Maniar HS, Schuessler RB, Damiano RJ Jr. Chronic transmural atrial ablation by using bipolar radiofrequency energy on the beating heart. The Journal of Thoracic and Cardiovascular Surgery. 2002;**124**(4):708-713

[35] Demaria RG, Page P, Leung TK, Dubuc M, Malo O, Carrier M, et al. Surgical radiofrequency ablation induces coronary endothelial dysfunction in porcine coronary arteries. European Journal of Cardio-Thoracic Surgery. 2003;**23**(3):277-282

[36] Gillinov AM, Pettersson G, Rice TW. Esophageal injury during radiofrequency ablation for atrial fibrillation. The Journal of Thoracic and Cardiovascular Surgery. 2001;**122**(6):1239-1240

[37] Gillinov AM, McCarthy PM, Pettersson G, Lytle BW, Rice TW. Esophageal perforation during left atrial radiofrequency ablation: Is the risk too high? The Journal of Thoracic and Cardiovascular Surgery. 2003;**126**(5):1661-1662

[38] Kottkamp H, Hindricks G, Autschbach R, Krauss B, Strasser B, S chirdewahn P, et al. Specific linear left atrial lesions in atrial fibrillation: Intraoperative radiofrequency ablation using minimally invasive surgical techniques. Journal of the American College of Cardiology. 2002;**40**(3):475-480

[39] Doll N, Borger MA, Fabricius A, Stephan S, Gummert J, Mohr FW, et al. Esophageal perforation during left atrial radiofrequency ablation: Is the risk too high? The Journal of Thoracic and Cardiovascular Surgery. 2003;**125**(4):836-842

[40] Saint LL, Lawrance CP, Okada S, Kazui T, Robertson JO, Schuessler RB, et al. Performance of a novel bipolar/monopolar radiofrequency ablation device on the beating heart in an acute porcine model. Innovations (Phila). 2013;**8**(4):276-283

[41] Groh MA, Binns OA, Burton HG 3rd, Champsaur GL, Ely SW, Johnson AM. Epicardial ultrasonic ablation of atrial fibrillation during concomitant cardiac surgery is a valid option in patients with ischemic heart disease. Circulation. 2008;**118**(14 Suppl):S78-S82

[42] Klinkenberg TJ, Ahmed S, Ten Hagen A, Wiesfeld AC, Tan ES, Zijlstra F, et al. Feasibility and outcome of epicardial pulmonary vein isolation for lone atrial fibrillation using minimal invasive surgery and high intensity focused ultrasound. Europace. 2009;**11**(12):1624-1631

[43] Mitnovetski S, Almeida AA, Goldstein J, Pick AW, Smith JA. Epicardial high-intensity focused ultrasound cardiac ablation for surgical treatment of atrial fibrillation. Heart, Lung & Circulation. 2009;**18**(1):28-31

[44] Nakagawa H, Antz M, Wong T, Schmidt B, Ernst S, Ouyang F, et al. Initial experience using a forward directed, high-intensity focused ultrasound balloon catheter for pulmonary vein antrum isolation in patients with atrial fibrillation. Journal of Cardiovascular Electrophysiology. 2007;**18**(2):136-144

[45] Ninet J, Roques X, Seitelberger R, Deville C, Pomar JL, Robin J, et al. Surgical ablation of atrial fibrillation with off-pump, epicardial, high-intensity focused ultrasound: Results of a multicenter trial. The Journal of Thoracic and Cardiovascular Surgery. 2005;**130**(3):803-809

[46] Kirchhof P, Benussi S, Kotecha D, Ahlsson A, Atar D, Casadei B, et al. ESC guidelines for the management of atrial fibrillation developed in collaboration with EACTS. Revista Espanola de Cardiologia. 2016, 2017;**70**(1):50

[47] Badhwar V, Rankin JS, Damiano RJ Jr, Gillinov AM, Bakaeen FG, Edgerton JR, et al. The Society of Thoracic Surgeons 2017 Clinical practice guidelines for the surgical treatment of atrial fibrillation. The Annals of Thoracic Surgery. 2017;**103**(1):329-341

[48] Weimar T, Bailey MS, Watanabe Y, Marin D, Maniar HS, Schuessler RB, et al. The Cox-maze IV procedure for lone atrial fibrillation: A single center experience in 100 consecutive patients. Journal of Interventional Cardiac Electrophysiology. 2011;**31**(1):47-54

[49] Lall SC, Melby SJ, Voeller RK, Zierer A, Bailey MS, Guthrie TJ, et al. The effect of ablation technology on surgical outcomes after the Cox-maze procedure: A propensity analysis. The Journal of Thoracic and Cardiovascular Surgery. 2007;**133**(2):389-396

[50] Lawrance CP, Henn MC, Damiano RJ Jr. Surgical ablation for atrial fibrillation: Techniques, indications, and results. Current Opinion in Cardiology. 2015;**30**(1):58-64

[51] Arcidi JM Jr, Doty DB, Millar RC. The Maze procedure: The LDS Hospital experience. Seminars in Thoracic and Cardiovascular Surgery. 2000;**12**(1):38-43

[52] Khiabani AJ, MacGregor RM, Bakir NH, Manghelli JL, Sinn LA, Maniar HS, et al. The long-term outcomes and durability of the Cox-Maze IV procedure for atrial fibrillation. The Journal of Thoracic and Cardiovascular Surgery. 2022;**163**(2):629-641

[53] Lawrance CP, Henn MC, Miller JR, Sinn LA, Schuessler RB, Maniar HS, et al. A minimally invasive Cox maze IV procedure is as effective as sternotomy while decreasing major morbidity and hospital stay. The Journal of Thoracic and Cardiovascular Surgery. 2014;**148**(3):955-961

[54] Ad N, Henry L, Friehling T, Wish M, Holmes SD. Minimally invasive stand-alone Cox-maze procedure for patients with nonparoxysmal atrial fibrillation.

The Annals of Thoracic Surgery. 2013;**96**(3):792-798

[55] Ad N, Holmes SD, Massimiano PS, Rongione AJ, Fornaresio LM. Long-term outcome following concomitant mitral valve surgery and Cox maze procedure for atrial fibrillation. The Journal of Thoracic and Cardiovascular Surgery. 2018;**155**(3):983-994

[56] Henn MC, Lancaster TS, Miller JR, Sinn LA, Schuessler RB, Moon MR, et al. Late outcomes after the Cox maze IV procedure for atrial fibrillation. The Journal of Thoracic and Cardiovascular Surgery. 2015;**150**(5):1168-1176

[57] Phan K, Xie A, Tsai YC, Kumar N, La Meir M, Yan TD. Biatrial ablation vs. left atrial concomitant surgical ablation for treatment of atrial fibrillation: A meta-analysis. Europace. 2015;**17**(1):38-47

[58] Gillinov AM, McCarthy PM, Blackstone EH, Rajeswaran J, Pettersson G, Sabik JF, et al. Surgical ablation of atrial fibrillation with bipolar radiofrequency as the primary modality. The Journal of Thoracic and Cardiovascular Surgery. 2005;**129**(6):1322-1329

[59] Voeller RK, Bailey MS, Zierer A, Lall SC, Sakamoto S, Aubuchon K, et al. Isolating the entire posterior left atrium improves surgical outcomes after the Cox maze procedure. The Journal of Thoracic and Cardiovascular Surgery. 2008;**135**(4):870-877

[60] Barnett SD, Ad N. Surgical ablation as treatment for the elimination of atrial fibrillation: A meta-analysis. The Journal of Thoracic and Cardiovascular Surgery. 2006;**131**(5):1029-1035

[61] Nitta T, Ishii Y, Miyagi Y, Ohmori H, Sakamoto S, Tanaka S. Concurrent multiple left atrial focal activations with fibrillatory conduction and right atrial focal or reentrant activation as the mechanism in atrial fibrillation. The Journal of Thoracic and Cardiovascular Surgery. 2004;**127**(3):770-778

[62] Sahadevan J, Ryu K, Peltz L, Khrestian CM, Stewart RW, Markowitz AH, et al. Epicardial mapping of chronic atrial fibrillation in patients: Preliminary observations. Circulation. 2004;**110**(21):3293-3299

[63] Schuessler RB, Kay MW, Melby SJ, Branham BH, Boineau JP, Damiano RJ. Spatial and temporal stability of the dominant frequency of activation in human atrial fibrillation. Journal of Electrocardiology. 2006;**39** (4 Suppl):S7-S12

[64] Haissaguerre M, Jais P, Shah DC, Takahashi A, Hocini M, Quiniou G, et al. Spontaneous initiation of atrial fibrillation by ectopic beats originating in the pulmonary veins. The New England Journal of Medicine. 1998;**339**(10):659-666

[65] Lee SH, Tai CT, Hsieh MH, Tsao HM, Lin YJ, Chang SL, et al. Predictors of non-pulmonary vein ectopic beats initiating paroxysmal atrial fibrillation: Implication for catheter ablation. Journal of the American College of Cardiology. 2005;**46**(6):1054-1059

[66] DeSimone CV, Noheria A, Lachman N, Edwards WD, Gami AS, Maleszewski JJ, et al. Myocardium of the superior vena cava, coronary sinus, vein of Marshall, and the pulmonary vein ostia: Gross anatomic studies in 620 hearts. Journal of Cardiovascular Electrophysiology. 2012;**23**(12):1304-1309

[67] Geuzebroek GS, Ballaux PK, van Hemel NM, Kelder JC, Defauw JJ. Medium-term outcome of different surgical methods to cure atrial

fibrillation: Is less worse? Interactive Cardiovascular and Thoracic Surgery. 2008;**7**(2):201-206

[68] Reyes G, Benedicto A, Bustamante J, Sarraj A, Nuche JM, Alvarez P, et al. Restoration of atrial contractility after surgical cryoablation: Clinical, electrical and mechanical results. Interactive Cardiovascular and Thoracic Surgery. 2009;**9**(4):609-612

[69] Pruitt JC, Lazzara RR, Dworkin GH, Badhwar V, Kuma C, Ebra G. Totally endoscopic ablation of lone atrial fibrillation: Initial clinical experience. The Annals of Thoracic Surgery. 2006;**81**(4):1325-1330

[70] Wolf RK, Schneeberger EW, Osterday R, Miller D, Merrill W, Flege JB Jr, et al. Video-assisted bilateral pulmonary vein isolation and left atrial appendage exclusion for atrial fibrillation. The Journal of Thoracic and Cardiovascular Surgery. 2005;**130**(3):797-802

[71] Boersma LV, Castella M, van Boven W, Berruezo A, Yilmaz A, Nadal M, et al. Atrial fibrillation catheter ablation versus surgical ablation treatment (FAST): A 2-center randomized clinical trial. Circulation. 2012;**125**(1):23-30

[72] Healey JS, Crystal E, Lamy A, Teoh K, Semelhago L, Hohnloser SH, et al. Left Atrial Appendage Occlusion Study (LAAOS): Results of a randomized controlled pilot study of left atrial appendage occlusion during coronary bypass surgery in patients at risk for stroke. American Heart Journal. 2005;**150**(2):288-293

[73] Salzberg SP, Gillinov AM, Anyanwu A, Castillo J, Filsoufi F, Adams DH. Surgical left atrial appendage occlusion: Evaluation of a novel device with magnetic resonance imaging. European Journal of Cardio-Thoracic Surgery. 2008;**34**(4):766-770

[74] Salzberg SP, Plass A, Emmert MY, Desbiolles L, Alkadhi H, Grunenfelder J, et al. Left atrial appendage clip occlusion: Early clinical results. The Journal of Thoracic and Cardiovascular Surgery. 2010;**139**(5):1269-1274

[75] Cuculich PS, Wang Y, Lindsay BD, Faddis MN, Schuessler RB, Damiano RJ Jr, et al. Noninvasive characterization of epicardial activation in humans with diverse atrial fibrillation patterns. Circulation. 2010;**122**(14):1364-1372

[76] Vijayakumar R, Ruaengsri C, et al. The arrhythmic substrate for atrial fibrillation in patients with mitral regurgitation. Journal of Atrial Fibrillation. 2020;**13**(2):2304

Chapter 11

Frozen Hearts: The Emerging Role of Cryoablation for Pulmonary Vein Isolation

Jonathan Tardos, Nawal Aamir, Dhaval Desai, Amanda Chajkowski and Amit H. Patel

Abstract

The cornerstone for the modern treatment of paroxysmal atrial fibrillation (AF) is pulmonary vein isolation, also called an AF ablation. Various ablation technologies exist to accomplish this goal with specific advantages. This chapter will focus on the unique attributes of cryoablation for pulmonary vein isolation. Specifically, we will summarize the trial data and outcomes of cryoablation in patients with paroxysmal and persistent AF from the initial FDA approval studies to novel uses beyond the pulmonary veins. Readers will have an appreciation of the unique characteristics differentiating cryoablation from radiofrequency (RF) catheter ablation and other techniques such as surgical MAZE. Clinical trial data show both noninferiority, and in some cases, superior outcomes of cryoablation to antiarrhythmic drug therapy and other ablation techniques.

Keywords: cryoablation, atrial fibrillation, ablation, pulmonary vein isolation, AF ablation

1. Introduction

Atrial fibrillation (AF) is the most common sustained arrhythmia in the United States. Symptoms vary widely, and can include: palpitations, dizziness, chest discomfort, fatigue, shortness of breath, and stroke [1]. There are many factors that can increase one's risk of developing AF which include: age, increased body mass index (BMI), hypertension (HTN), diabetes mellitus (DM), congestive heart failure (CHF), obstructive sleep apnea (OSA), and some genetic predispositions as well. In addition to these risk factors, certain lifestyle characteristics can also play a role in the development or perpetuation of AF. These factors include smoking, alcohol, and psychosocial stress [2].

For patients with AF, the two principal goals of long-term therapy are to improve quality of life (e.g., symptom control) and to prevent associated morbidity and mortality. Rate and rhythm control strategies both can improve symptoms, but interestingly, neither has been conclusively shown to improve survival compared to the other. For those patients in whom a rhythm control strategy is chosen, catheter ablation or antiarrhythmic drugs are the two principal therapeutic options. This chapter will review the efficacy and safety of these two options for rhythm control and provides rationale for choosing one versus the other [3].

The incidence and prevalence of AF has been increasing globally. Data from the Framingham Heart Study demonstrated that the prevalence of AF increased 3-fold over the past 50 years [4]. The prevalence of AF doubles with every decade of life and reaches close to 9% in the ninth decade. In 2019, AF was mentioned on over 180,000 death certificates and was the underlying cause of death in approximately 15% of those deaths. According to the CDC, it is estimated that more than 12.1 million individuals in the United States will have AF in 2030. The worldwide prevalence of AF was approximately 46.3 million individuals in 2016 [5]. In Europe, the prevalence of AF in 2010 was 9 million among people older than 55 years and is expected to reach around 14 million by 2060 [6].

Clinically, AF can be classified by the duration of episodes and responsiveness to therapies as follows:

1. Paroxysmal AF (PAF) is characterized as self-limited episodes of AF typically separated widely, with no episode lasting greater than seven days.

2. Persistent AF, which is characterized by AF that is present for more than seven days or with a need for intervention to resume sinus rhythm (chemical or electrical cardioversion).

3. Permanent AF, where cardioversion is either not effective, or sinus rhythm reverts back to AF immediately.

AF is a complex process that results in rapid and disorganized atrial activation. Understanding the mechanisms of AF helps to understand the rationale behind the therapeutic interventions. The triggers for AF episodes most commonly are premature atrial contractions (PAC) which originate from within the pulmonary veins (PVs). Increased time in AF leads to structural changes throughout the atria such as scarring and fibrosis. These changes decrease the likelihood of spontaneous conversion to normal sinus rhythm (NSR) in patients with persistent or permanent AF [2, 7, 8].

The goal in circumferential pulmonary vein isolation (PVI) is to electrically separate the left atrium from the source of the PAC foci within the pulmonary veins. Circumferential pulmonary vein ablation has several putative mechanisms of action and is the mainstay for ablative treatments for AF. Other mechanisms by which circumferential ablation is believed to be effective are by concomitant ablation of the autonomic ganglia, which are found near the pulmonary vein ostia. Circumferential ablation is typically recommended for patients with PAF; however, it can also be beneficial for patients with persistent AF alone or in combination with additional ablation sites.

2. Catheter ablation vs. antiarrhythmic drugs

For patients with either paroxysmal or persistent AF who desire sinus rhythm, catheter ablation or long-term antiarrhythmic drug therapy are the two available approaches. There are defined risks and benefits to the different approaches. This section will review the studies that have directly compared them. It is important to note that this section is not intended to address management of patients who have failed rhythm control with two or more antiarrhythmic drugs or those who have already received catheter ablation. Antiarrhythmic drug therapy failure is defined as a trial of a drug that results in reduction in AF burden that is not satisfactory to the patient, or results in side effects that are intolerable to the patient, proarrhythmic, or result in organ toxicity [9, 10]. Prior to the 2020 ACC / AHA / HRS guidelines, catheter ablation (CA) was generally recommended as second line therapy after failure of AADs. However, mounting evidence suggested that CA is superior to AAD for the control of symptoms and maintenance of NSR. CA is now accepted as a first-line therapy for symptomatic patients after a comprehensive discussion of the benefits and risks of both approaches [3, 11].

Typically, evaluation of the various AF treatment strategies includes reference to the time free of AF in the year following treatment initiation. This is commonly referred to as the 1 year AF free survival. The 1 year data commonly excludes the 90-day blanking period following treatment to allow for post-ablation healing. An AF free survival of 100% would mean no patients had AF recurrences, and 0% 1 year AF free survival would mean all patients studied had recurrence within a year. Three early meta-analyses of studies comparing catheter ablation and antiarrhythmic drug therapy found that AF free survival was higher in the ablation treatment arm as compared to the AAD treatment arm [12, 13]. In the EARLY-AF trial, 303 patients were assigned to either AAD group (n = 149) or cryoablation group (n = 154). All the patients in both groups received an implantable cardiac monitoring device to assess AF recurrences and the follow-up period was 12 months. The first documented atrial tachyarrhythmia included for analysis had to occur between 91 and 365 days after CA or AAD initiation. The AF free survival was 89% of patients who underwent CA and 74% of the patients who were started on AAD (hazard ratio, 0.39; 95% CI, 0.22 to 0.68) [14]. Another study demonstrated similar results, which reported an 1-year AF free survival of 58% of patients undergoing CA and 32% of patients assigned to AAD therapy (hazard ratio, 0.48; 95% confidence interval [CI], 0.35 to 0.66; $P < 0.001$) [15]. In another trial that included 203 patients, 104 underwent CA and 99 received AAD therapy. In the ablation group, the procedure had initial success in 97% of the patients. The 1 year AF free survival was 74.6% (95% confidence interval, 65.0 to 82.0) in the ablation group and 45.0% (95% CI, 34.6 to 54.7) in the drug-therapy group ($P < 0.001$) [16, 17].

Important complications of AF ablations include cardiac tamponade (about 1%), pulmonary vein stenosis (<1%), phrenic nerve paralysis (~ 3%with cryoballoon), and rare instances of stroke and atrioesophageal fistula. Of the 303 patients in EARLY-AF, serious adverse events occurred in 5 patients in the CA group (3.2%) and in 6 patients (4%) of patients in the AAD group. Commonly prescribed drugs to maintain sinus rhythm are amiodarone, sotalol, dofetilide, dronedarone, flecainide, and propafenone. These medications range in efficacy from 40 to 60% 1 year AF free survival in meta-analyses. Important AAD medication side effects include proarrhythmia, bradyarrhythmia, organ toxicity, and death [17]. AAD selection is influenced by the patient's comorbid conditions such as CHF, CAD, structural heart disease, kidney function, and liver function. Guidelines exist to help in the selection of the appropriate agents with these comorbid conditions in mind to minimize potential drug toxicities and side effects. However, the guideline adherence when prescribing these medications is poor [18]. Importantly, all patients need to be informed of the possibility of recurrence of AF and adverse events with both catheter and medication-based rhythm control strategies.

Evaluating RF ablation versus AAD, the ThermoCool AF study randomly assigned 167 symptomatic patients with PAF who failed at least one AAD and who experienced at least three episodes of paroxysmal AF within the six months prior to randomization to either catheter ablation (with RF) or AAD therapy. Patients with significant left ventricular dysfunction, persistent AF, and advanced heart failure were excluded. Catheter ablation included PVI with confirmation of entrance block, and AAD therapy included flecainide (36 percent), propafenone (41 percent), dofetilide, sotalol, or quinidine at the investigator's discretion. After nine months, there were significantly fewer patients with documented symptomatic paroxysmal AF in the catheter ablation group (84 versus 34 percent AF free survival; hazard ratio 0.30, 95% CI 0.19–0.47). In addition, major treatment-related adverse events occurred more often with AAD therapy (9 versus 5 percent) at 30 days. Mean quality-of-life scores improved significantly with catheter ablation compared to AAD therapy [19].

A similar trial to ThermoCool AF was conducted for the cryoballoon catheter. The STOP AF trial is an important trial that specifically studied the use of AADs versus CA in patients with PAF. There were a total of 245 patients studied, all with either a diagnosis of PAF or persistent AF. All the patients included in the study had a history of previous AAD failure. In the AAD group, patients were randomly assigned to flecainide, propafenone, or sotalol. A "blanking period" was used in this study, which essentially allowed for medical optimization of any AAD or necessary re-ablation in the CA group. Treatment success was defined as the freedom from any detectable AF after the blanking period. The patients in both the experimental groups were followed for twelve months following intervention. Among those in the AAD group, 78% with PAF and 22% with persistent AF experienced failure of at least one AAD. On the other hand, 98.2% of patients in the CA group achieved acute isolation in three or more of the PVs, and 97.6% in all four PVs. A 1-year AF-free survival was found in 69.9% of CA patients, and 7.3% of patients in the AAD group. Among those patients who underwent CA, symptoms were significantly improved at the twelve-month mark as well [20].

The Catheter Ablation vs. Antiarrhythmic Drug Therapy in Atrial Fibrillation (CABANA) trial was a more recent large clinical trial looking at catheter ablation versus AAD in patients with AF. This study also evaluated patients with either paroxysmal (43%) or persistent AF (57%) and randomly assigned each patient to either AAD or CA therapy. Patients were excluded from the study if they had any prior catheter ablation procedure or failure of two or more antiarrhythmic drugs. It is important to note that in this study, of the patients who received AAD drug therapy, 27.5% crossed over to the ablation group. The primary endpoint of this study was death, disabling stroke, serious bleeding or cardiac arrest, which occurred in 8.0 and 9.2% in the AAD and CA groups, respectively during the 4 year follow up period. There was no significant difference in all-cause mortality (5.2% vs. 6.1%) among both respective groups. The trial showed that the combined end point of death or cardiovascular hospitalization occurred less often among those who underwent CA as it did for recurrence of AF. The quality of life scores for each group showed significant improvement. However, those in the CA group reported significantly greater improvement than the drug therapy group at twelve months with scores of 86.4 and 80.9 points, respectively, with a baseline reference value of 63 points [21].

To further assess the efficacy and safety of CA as compared to AADs as first line treatment for PAF, a meta-analysis was conducted of six studies that compared CA with AAD. Among studies in the meta-analysis, a total of 1200 patients were included. Catheter ablation was associated with lower rates of recurrent atrial arrhythmias consistently. The risks of serious adverse events, including stroke, cardiac tamponade, and death were also evaluated. It was demonstrated that lower rates of symptomatic atrial arrhythmias, lower healthcare resource utilization, and lower rates of crossover to alternative treatment were all associated with first line CA strategy. However, this particular meta-analysis did have limitations which included a moderate degree of heterogeneity among the included studies most notably the RAAFT 2 trial [22].

The CASTLE AF trial demonstrated improved outcomes with upfront ablation among patients with chronic systolic congestive heart failure who are otherwise receiving appropriate treatment [21]. CASTLE AF used implantable cardioverter defibrillators equipped with AF monitoring capabilities to study AF recurrences in patients after randomization to initial catheter ablation or AAD therapy. Patients were excluded if they had a prior history of daily use of class I or class III antiarrhythmic drugs. The primary endpoint was considered to be death or hospitalization for worsening heart failure, and this was demonstrated in significantly fewer patients in the CA group in comparison to the AAD group. After a 60 month follow up period, 63.1% of the patients in the CA group and 21.7% of patients in the AAD group remained in sinus rhythm. In other words, the CA patients had a significantly lower recurrence of AF than those in the AAD group. In terms of mortality, fewer patients in the ablation group (28.5%) in comparison to the AAD group (44.6%) experienced the primary endpoint of death from any cause [10, 23].

In summary, CA is useful for symptomatic paroxysmal AF as a first line therapy when a rhythm control strategy is desired. Catheter ablation for AF is safe and effective with similar or improved outcomes as compared to AADs for long term AF management with fewer long-term complications. Upfront catheter ablation as noted in the CASTLE-AF trial is associated with reductions in all-cause mortality in patients with CHF. A discussion with patients regarding these risks and benefits should guide decisions on which strategy to utilize in the maintenance of normal sinus rhythm (NSR).

3. Cryoablation vs. radiofrequency

Catheter ablation is now a well-established interventional approach for treating symptomatic, drug refractory PAF with class I level A guidelines recommendation. A 2017 randomized comparison between cryoablation and RFA showed similar success rates, as did a meta-analysis of observational studies. Historically, catheter ablation using either cryoablation or radiofrequency ablation demonstrated 60–80% 1 year AF free survival.

Cryoablation for arrhythmias has been used for cardiac surgery for decades. However, transvenous catheter cryoablation for arrhythmias have been used only since the 2000s. The main purpose of cryoballoon ablation (CBA) is to isolate pulmonary veins (PVs) with single energy application for encircling lesions at the antral level of the PVs. Conventional radiofrequency catheter ablation (RF) was characterized by point-by-point ablation to create a line which requires multiple energy applications to accomplish PVI [24].

The procedure of cryoablation is performed in the cardiac catheterization / electrophysiology laboratory. Access is typically obtained through the right femoral vein. Additional access is often required from the left femoral vein and/or the axillary or internal jugular vein depending on the operator's preference. The ablation technique for cryoballoon ablation is similar to that of radiofrequency ablation in that a septal puncture is used to access the left atrium with the goal of PVI. In the case of cryoablation, only a single transseptal puncture is required though at a lower anterior septal location. This location is recommended to allow more space for the cryoballoon to move and provide better support to the PVs, especially the right inferior PV [10].

With the assistance of fluoroscopy, and 3D electroanatomical mapping technologies including intracardiac echocardiography; transseptal puncture is performed to gain access to the left atrium. The ablation can be made in any sequence, but it is commonly started with the left superior pulmonary vein then left inferior pulmonary vein followed by the right inferior pulmonary vein and finally the right superior pulmonary vein [1]. Esophageal temperature monitoring is frequently performed to avoid potentially dangerous cooling of the esophagus during adjacent LA cryoablation. Similarly, the right phrenic nerve is paced during right-sided pulmonary vein applications to avoid phrenic nerve damage. After ablation is completed, a mapping catheter is placed into each pulmonary vein to check for proper electrical isolation. A vein is considered acutely isolated if it demonstrates entrance and exit electrical block [25].

Radiofrequency is completed using a current which is applied in a point-by-point method. The resistive current allows for the tissue to be heated, and this results in cellular necrosis. Alternatively, the use of cryothermal energy, which is applied with a balloon, differs from the former as it allows for cellular necrosis via freezing [24]. Cryoballoon technology is increasingly used for treating AF. Although commonly there are 2 right-sided and 2 left-sided pulmonary veins, there are frequently noted anatomical variants. Cryoballoon ablation for PAF was associated with similar clinical outcomes as radiofrequency independently of the anatomical pulmonary vein distribution pattern. The presence of a left common ostium or right middle vein was found to have similar clinical outcomes after cryoablation when compared with a control group treated by standard radiofrequency ablation. Pulmonary vein anatomical variants should not influence the choice of cryoballoon ablation [26].

There are many studies that compare the efficacy of cryoballoon ablation to radiofrequency, and a few of those trials have been outlined below. However, it is important to note that many of these studies involve relatively small sample sizes which are accompanied by a number of confounding variables. Systematic literature reviews and meta-analysis evaluating efficacy of cryoablation versus radiofrequency ablation for treating paroxysmal AF are helpful to make comparisons in this light [10, 26]. In a meta-analysis by Yi-He Chen et al., of 273 scholarly articles containing comparison between radiofrequency ablation and cryoablation of PAF. There were a total of 7195 participants studied, approximately one third (2863) underwent cryoablation and two thirds (4332) underwent RF ablation. The mean age of the patients was 59.9 years old, with a history of PAF ranging from 2.1 to 5.2 years. The study types included were retrospective cohort and prospective cohort with one study being ambi-directional. Cryoablation of the pulmonary vein was performed with a second generation cryoballoon within the majority of the studies. The mean follow-up duration ranged from 12 to 18 months. There is no evidence of significant differences for patient baseline demographic characteristics between the CA and RF ablation groups [26]. The overall freedom from AF/atrial tachycardia relapse was 65.6% with CA and 60.1% with RF ablation in follow-up of 12 months. The pooled estimate of relative risk ratio indicated that PVI was achieved by CA and RF ablation, which lead to comparable long-term AF/atrial tachycardia free survival during follow-up. Relative risk was 1.05 with a 95% confidence interval of 0.98–1.13, $P = 0.159$. There were no statistically significant interactions between the pooled RR and prespecified covariants. Data on procedure related adverse events were available for meta-analysis in 15 studies. Events occurred in 223 of 2759 patients (8.08%) with cryoablation and 333 of 4130 patients (8.06%) with RF ablation. No significant difference was found between these 2 approaches for ablation procedure-related adverse events [26].

The *FIRE AND ICE* trial, the largest prospective multicenter comparison between the two techniques, demonstrated that the cryoballoon is noninferior to radiofrequency ablation (RFA) in efficacy. The primary efficacy endpoint was defined as the first documented clinical failure (recurrence of AF, episodes of atrial flutter, start of antiarrhythmic agent, or repeat ablation). The study also demonstrated no significant difference with regards to overall safety. There were no reports of deaths, esophageal fistulas, or pulmonary vein stenosis. With regards to concerns about phrenic nerve injury the study showed only 1 in 300 patients developed permanent phrenic nerve injury at 12 months.

There was no significant difference in fluoroscopy time between the 2 approaches but overall procedure time in CBA was significantly less. This is due to the fact that CBA is a 1-shot catheter rather than the point-by-point approach in RF ablation to achieve pulmonary vein isolation. The point-by-point RF mapping has a more complex learning curve as it requires great skill and is more technical than CBA. This is what is making CBA one of the most widely used catheter techniques.

RF ablation results in irreversible tissue damage via heating. In CA, the freezing process involves ice crystal formation. This allows for an osmotic gradient to develop, which subsequently leads to acute cell death. This mechanism of cell death involves cellular swelling and disruption of the membrane integrity by means of further osmotic insult. The histopathological features of CA may be responsible for relatively demarcated lesions with minimal tissue architectural disruption. This has been found to contribute to a lower risk of thrombus formation and perforation. In addition, cryoballoon CA has also demonstrated catheter adhesion to pulmonary vein (through freezing) and thus the prevention of dislodgement [27, 28].

The long-term freedom from AF at 12-month follow-up and overall postoperative complication rates is also important to evaluate. One meta-analysis reviewed 247 articles, with a total of 8 studies encompassing 1548 patients who underwent either cryoballoon or radiofrequency ablation. This is representative of data from Europe between 2012 and 2015. Overall, it was found there is no significant difference between the freedom from AF after 12 months between both groups cryoballoon and radiofrequency ablation. Secondary outcomes during the ablation at the fluoroscopy time the ablation time failed to reach significance as well. Cryoablation had a significantly greater odds of postop phrenic nerve injury after 12 months [29].

A novel way of comparing the effectiveness of cryoballoon ablation and radiofrequency ablation was demonstrated by Trippoli et al. with a pooling method referred to as the Shiny method. The Shiny method is based on an artificial intelligence that reconstructs individual patient data. Using the Shiny method is unique because it accounts for follow-up length. This method was used for reevaluation of a meta-analysis. The advantage to using this method in re-analysis is because researchers are able to evaluate the probability of the end-point in the long term. The primary endpoint was time to recurrence of AF in patients who were enrolled in randomized studies comparing CA to AAD, RF to AAD, and CA to RF. Overall, CA showed a statistically significant higher effectiveness than AAD therapy. In the comparison of AAD to RF, no statistically significant difference was observed. This suggests that the results generated by the Shiny method from previously published meta-analysis were able to account for the effects of randomizations performed in the trials, along with accounting for length of follow up in the individual trials [30].

Atrial esophageal fistula is a well described complication of RF ablation where an abnormal potentially life-threatening connection forms between the esophagus and right atrium by a mis-match repair mechanism. It is hypothesized that this occurs due to inflammation caused by energy delivery to the posterior wall of the left atrium adjacent to the esophagus. Although initially believed to be a unique complication related to RF ablation, cryoablation has also been associated with this potentially fatal complication though far less frequently. A study by Ripley et al. dives further into the adverse effect of esophageal lesions after catheter ablation with cryoballoon and RF ablation and the implication for atrial esophageal fistula formation. The effects of direct application of RF and cryoablation on the cervical esophagus were evaluated in 16 calves. Cryoablation was performed with a 6.5 mm catheter probe using a single 5-minute freeze at less than −80°C. RF ablation was delivered with an 8 mm catheter electrode at 50 W and 50°C for 45 to 60 seconds. Histopathological assessments were performed at 1, 4, 7, and 14 days after the completion of both ablation procedures. This article evaluated the direct application of cryoablation and RF ablation in the left atrium and its effects on the esophagus. Although, on day 14 lesions in both groups on the esophagus were comparable in size, there was histological evidence of partial to full wall esophageal lesion ulceration associated with 0 of 44 cryoablation lesions and in 9 of the 41 lesions with RF ablation (P equals 0.0025). In other words, Cryoablation was associated with a significantly lower risk of esophageal ulceration [30].

4. Cryoballoon evolution

RF ablation catheters have made advancements over the years but they still rely on a "point-by-point" technique to achieve PVI which can be challenging and time-consuming. This is due to the fact that RF ablation utilizes focal catheters as opposed to a balloon system that can produce circumferential continuous lesions resulting in shorter TTI and durable PVI.

The Arctic Front™ is the first cryoballoon catheter system introduced in the United States, and was used in the North American STOP AF trial. The study found that the first generation CB was a safe and effective alternative to antiarrhythmic therapy. Procedure times were sped up to about one third when compared to spot ablation techniques.

Evolution of CB from first to the second-generation included the addition of 4 jets, increased refrigerant flow, and moving the cooling zone more distally. These changes made the CB more efficacious. The second generation CB was used in the FIRE and ICE trial that demonstrated Cryoablation to be noninferior to RF ablation.

The latest technological advances in the family of CB include improved visualization of TTI and maneuverability of the catheter. Further modifications are inevitable and will surely provide even safer and more efficient catheters [31, 32].

5. Stereotaxis

Guiding the catheter to the intended sites and maintaining adequate contact is a critical part of a successful procedure. The ability to see left atrium anatomy reduces complications and ensures that lesions are made at intended target sites.

Fluoroscopy was the main imaging technique used by electrophysiologists to target the ablation site however it had several drawbacks including 2-dimensional (2-D) representation, inability to visualize soft tissue, and a long learning curve. Other modalities to facilitate accessing the left atrium anatomy include intracardiac echocardiogram, computed tomography (CT) and magnetic resonance imaging (MRI).

Remote magnetic navigation (Stereotaxis) entered clinical use for electrophysiology interventional procedures several years ago. Using stereotaxis may help reduce the risk of complications and increase the patient's safety. The system creates a weak magnetic field around the patient that can be manipulated by an integrated computer and three-dimensional mapping system to drive flexible catheters within the heart with extreme precision.

Over the past 10 years, AF ablation has become the predominant indication in centers of excellence, possibly representing up to 60% of interventions. The main difficulties during these procedures are the duration, which may exceed 4 hours, and the length of time that both the operator and patient are exposed to radiation. The advantages of the technique were underlined by different authors, who highlighted that there was no risk of perforation, the catheter had excellent stability, and it was possible to navigate in complex anatomies, as has been described in patients with congenital heart defects. Although AF ablation was noticeably effective in 80% of cases, with a mean of 1.3–1.7 procedures per patient, the rate of major complications reported was 4.5% of cases, including 1% vascular accidents and 1.3% tamponade [33].

Several clinical trials have now been undertaken to evaluate RMNS in AF. The initial phase evaluated the feasibility of RMNS in 40 AF patients who required treatment by RFA. The authors demonstrated the feasibility and very good efficacy of the robotic technique. Application time was significantly reduced compared with the control group, although the trial was a case-control study.9. The operator highlighted the extreme stability of the magnetic catheter, which was especially useful for approaching the right veins. In the study, success was achieved in 38 of the 40 patients tested (95% of cases) [34].

6. Other ablation strategies

Beyond minimally invasive strategies, there are surgical ablation techniques most well known of which is the COX-MAZE (CM) procedure. Surgical approaches to AF ablation vary in the technique and level of published research investigating outcomes. With changes in the goals of the procedure the CM has been revised multiple times with each interaction being assigned a roman numeral. The CM IV procedure had significantly shorter mean aortic cross-clamp time for a lone CM from 93 ± 34 min for the CM III to 47 ± 26 min for the CM IV ($P < 0.001$). A propensity analysis performed by Lall et al. showed no significant difference in freedom from AF at 3, 6 and 12 months postoperatively between appropriately matched patients undergoing either the CM III or the CM IV [34]. A report of over 2 decades by Weimar et al. demonstrated both the CM III and CM IV showed no difference in freedom from AF and a significantly decreased major complication rate. This was despite the fact that the recent cohort had more patients with long-standing persistent AF and much more intensive follow-up with the majority of patients having at least 24-h Holter monitoring [34].

A more recent CM IV study reviewed 576 consecutive patients who underwent the CM IV between January 2002 and September 2014. Most patients were followed up with prolonged Holter monitoring. Twelve-month freedom from AF was 93%, with 85% of patients free from all AADs, while 5-year freedom from AF was 78%, with 66% of patients also free from all AADs. When comparing patients with PAF to patients with persistent AF, freedom from AF on and off AADs was not significantly different at any time point [35].

The CM has been successful in reducing the incidence of stroke. In a report by Pet et al., 13% of the patients had experienced a preoperative neurological event out of the 433 studied. However, there were only 6 postoperative neurological events during long-term follow-up in this cohort (mean 6.6 ± 5.0 years). The long-term stroke rate after the CM has been 0.2% per year, despite the fact that the great majority of patients had discontinued AADs [36].

Other cardiac diseases are often seen along with AF, and the CM is commonly used as an associated procedure. In patients who underwent mitral valve surgery, studies have demonstrated similar arrhythmia recurrence rates in patients with lone AF who have undergone stand-alone surgical ablation compared to those with AF and mitral regurgitation who underwent concomitant mitral procedures. Specifically, freedom from AF and AADs at 12 and 24 months were nearly the same between the 2 groups (73% vs. 76% at 12 months, 77% vs. 78% at 24 months) [37]. Another prospective, randomized control trial which was performed at the Cardiothoracic Surgical Trials Network (CTSN) compared patients with persistent or long -standing AF with patients who had mitral valve disease that required surgical intervention. The experimental groups either underwent CA or no ablation. The results demonstrated that the patients that remained free from AF at both 6 and 12 months belonged to that of the CA group with $P < 0.001$. It is important to note that those patients that underwent CA did not significantly affect morbidity or mortality.

A comparison between patients undergoing stand-alone CM-IV to those undergoing CA with aortic valve replacement was just as effective as stone-alone CM IV in the treatment of AF among all ages and all comorbidities [38]. Outcomes of patients with AF that were planning on having left or biatrial CM IV and coronary artery bypass grafting (CABG) in the years of 2002 to 2015 demonstrated significantly low operative mortality rates. Freedom from AF at 1 year in the CM-IV group was upwards of 98% with 88% free of AADs at the 5 year follow up period [35–38].

Minimally invasive right minithoracotomy (RMT) is an alternate approach to standard surgical sternotomy approach. RMT has been associated with reduced operative morbidity and decreased intensive care unit stays. Major surgical complications were also found to be significantly lower in the RMT groups in composition to standard surgical approach [39].

In the last 3 decades, the development of ablation technologies has positively impacted the field of AF surgery and patient outcomes. Minimally invasive technologies have decreased the need for CABG procedure time, and with minimally invasive technologies come improved morbidity and mortality for patients. The number of patients undergoing surgical ablation procedures has been vastly increasing in the past 2–3 decades; however, there are still a significant number of patients with AF that are undergoing other cardiac interventions without treatment for their AF. With increased research and knowledge, increased education can encourage more aggressive treatment of AF in these patients. As continued learning of AF and the mechanisms of which it can develop evolves, improved diagnostic technologies can be implemented to a larger volume of patients [40].

7. Alternate uses/future directions

Based on this biophysical characteristic of preserving the tissue architecture, cryoablation was preferred to reduce the risk of causing destruction to the normal structure during specific arrhythmias such as atrioventricular nodal reentrant tachycardia or tachycardia originating near the His bundle region. These characteristics explain the lower risk of cardiac perforation or thrombogenicity compared to RFA. Cryothermal energy is produced during refrigerants injected through a fine tube. The refrigerant vaporizes at the tip of a cryoablation catheter and can freeze the adjacent tissue. While freezing, the catheter tip adheres to the affected tissue, which enables the application of stable energy [41].

A high cooling power and culture with culture cryoablation also called Adagio combination of newly exploited cryogenically interchangeable stylette needles. Flexible continuous leak and creation of other tachyarrhythmia by optimizing her catheter shape. Patients who underwent AF ablation enrolled in this procedure in the assessment of the procedural data that was focused on safety comprising first-pass isolation and defined as a successful PVI after initial application. The studies follow sequential PV isolation using the Novell UL TC catheters to visit without compromising safety the first-pass isolation was accomplished about half of the PVs.

8. Conclusions

The cornerstone for the modern treatment of paroxysmal atrial fibrillation (AF) is pulmonary vein isolation, also called an AF ablation. Various ablation technologies exist to accomplish this goal with specific advantages. Upfront ablation strategies have been shown superior to AAD in certain patient populations. One unique ablation technology for pulmonary vein isolation is Cryoablation. Clinical trial data shows both non-inferiority, and in some cases, superior outcomes of cryoablation to antiarrhythmic drug therapy and other ablation techniques. Cryoablation has been shown to be safe, and effective in various common anatomic configurations. An evolving technology, newer generation cryoballoons offer improved efficacy and continued safety.

Acknowledgements

We would like to acknowledge and thank Community Medical Center for the support of the program and in specific, Jagan Vanjarapu MD and Nelson Okoh MD.

Thank you/notes

Thank you to our supportive families without which none of this would exist.

Appendices and nomenclature

AF	Atrial Fibrillation
BMI	Body Mass Index

HTN	Hypertension
DM	Diabetes Mellitus
HF	Heart Failure
OSA	Obstructive Sleep Apnea
PAF	Paroxysmal Atrial Fibrillation
AAD	Anti Arrhythmic drugs
CA	Cryoablation
RF	Radiofrequency
PNP	Phrenic Nerve Palsy
PVI	Pulmonary Vein Isolation
RMNS	Remote Magnetic Navigation System
AV	atrioventricular
RFA	Radio Frequency Ablation
CM	Cryo Generation
CABG	Coronary Artery Bypass Grafting
RMT	Minimally invasive right minithoracotomy
CB-1	First generation cryoballoon
CB-2	Second generation cryoballoon
cryo-AF	Cryoablation of AF

Author details

Jonathan Tardos[1*], Nawal Aamir[2], Dhaval Desai[3], Amanda Chajkowski[2] and Amit H. Patel[4]

1 Robert Wood Johnson University Hospital, New Brunswick, NJ, USA

2 Rutgers Health Community Medical Center, USA

3 Jersey Shore University Medical Center, Neptune, NJ, USA

4 Community Medical Center Toms River, USA

*Address all correspondence to: jonathantardos@gmail.com

References

[1] Marine JE. Catheter ablation therapy for supraventricular arrhythmias. Journal of the American Medical Association. 2007;**298**(23):2768-2778

[2] Staerk L, Sherer JA, Ko D, Benjamin EJ, Helm RH. Atrial fibrillation: Epidemiology, pathophysiology, and clinical outcomes. Circulation Research. 2017;**120**:1501-1517. DOI: 10.1161/CIRCRESAHA.117.309732

[3] Andrade JG, Champagne J, Dubuc M, Deyell MW, Verma A, Macle L, et al. Cryoballoon or radiofrequency ablation for atrial fibrillation assessed by continuous monitoring: A Randomized Clinical Trial. Circulation. 2019;**140**(22):1779

[4] Lip GY, Beevers DG. ABC of atrial fibrillation. History, epidemiology, and importance of atrial fibrillation. BMJ. 1995;**311**:1361-1363

[5] Benjamin EJ, Muntner P, Alonso A, Bittencourt MS, Callaway CW, Carson AP, et al. American Heart Association Council on epidemiology and prevention statistics committee and stroke statistics subcommittee. Heart disease and stroke Statistics-2019 update: A report from the American Heart Association. Circulation. 2019;**139**:e56-e528

[6] Kannel WB, Benjamin EJ. Status of the epidemiology of atrial fibrillation. The Medical Clinics of North America. 2008;**92**(1):17

[7] Kornej J, Börschel CS, Benjamin EJ, Schnabel RB. Epidemiology of Atrial Fibrillation in the 21st Century. Circulation Research. 2020;**127**(1):4-20. DOI: 10.1161/circresaha.120.316340

[8] Lloyd-Jones DM, Wang TJ, Leip EP, Larson MG, Levy D, Vasan RS, et al. Lifetime risk for development of atrial fibrillation: The Framingham Heart Study. Circulation. 31 Aug 2004;**110**(9):1042-1046. DOI: 10.1161/01.CIR.0000140263.20897.42. Epub 2004 Aug 16. PMID: 15313941

[9] Andrade J, Khairy P, Dobrev D, Nattel S. The clinical profile and pathophysiology of atrial fibrillation: Relationships among clinical features, epidemiology, and mechanisms. Circulation Research. 2014;**114**(9):1453-1468

[10] Jin ES, Wang PJ. Cryoballoon ablation for atrial fibrillation: A comprehensive review and practice guide. Korean Circulation Journal. 2018;**48**(2):114-123. DOI: 10.4070/kcj.2017.0318

[11] Camm AJ et al. Guidelines for the management of atrial fibrillation: The Task Force for the Management of Atrial Fibrillation of the European Society of Cardiology (ESC). European Heart Journal. 2010;**31**:2369

[12] Chen HS, Wen JM, Wu SN, Liu JP. Catheter ablation for paroxysmal and persistent atrial fibrillation. Cochrane Database System Review. Apr 2012;**18**(4):CD007101. DOI: 10.1002/14651858.CD007101.pub2. PMID: 22513945

[13] Samuel M, Almohammadi M, Tsadok MA, et al. Population-Based Evaluation of Major Adverse Events After Catheter Ablation for Atrial Fibrillation. JACC Clinical Electrophysiology. 2017;**3**:1425

[14] Whittaker DK. Mechanisms of tissue destruction following cryosurgery.

Annals of the Royal College of Surgeons in England. 1984;**66**(5):313

[15] Oussama M. Wazni, Gopi Dandamudi, Nitesh Sood, Robert Hoyt, Jaret Tyler, Sarfraz Durrani, Mark Niebauer, Kevin Makati, Blair Halperin, Andre Gauri, Gustavo Morales, Mingyuan Shao, et al., Cryoballoon Ablation as Initial Therapy for Atrial Fibrillation

[16] Noheria A, Kumar A, Wylie JV, Josephson ME. Catheter ablation vs antiarrhythmic drug therapy for atrial fibrillation: A systematic review. Archives of Internal Medicine. 2008;**168**(6):581

[17] Terasawa T, Balk EM, Chung M, Garlitski AC, Alsheikh-Ali AA, Lau J, et al. Systematic review: Comparative effectiveness of radiofrequency catheter ablation for atrial fibrillation. Internal Medicine. 2009;**151**(3):191

[18] Tardos JG, Ronk CJ, Patel MY, Koren A, Kim MH. US antiarrhythmic drug treatment for patients with atrial fibrillation: An insurance claims–based report. Journal of the American Heart Association. 2021;**10**(6):e016792

[19] Wilber DJ, Pappone C, Neuzil P, De Paola A, Marchlinski F, Natale A, Macle L, Daoud EG, Calkins H, Hall B, Reddy V, Augello G, Reynolds MR. Comparison of antiarrhythmic drug therapy and radiofrequency catheter ablation in patients with paroxysmal atrial fibrillation: A randomized controlled trial

[20] Packer DL, Kowal RC, Wheelan KR, Irwin JM, Champagne J, Guerra PG, et al. Cryoballoon ablation of pulmonary veins for paroxysmal atrial fibrillation: First results of the north American Arctic front (STOP AF) pivotal trial. Journal of the American College of Cardiology. 2013;**61**(16):1713-1723

[21] Packer DL, Mark DB, Robb RA, Monahan KH, Bahnson TD, Poole JE, et al. Effect of catheter ablation vs antiarrhythmic drug therapy on mortality, stroke, bleeding, and cardiac arrest among patients with atrial fibrillation: The CABANA Randomized Clinical Trial. Journal of the American Medical Association. 2019;**321**(13):126

[22] Imberti JF, Ding WY, Kotalczyk A, Zhang J, Boriani G, Lip G, et al. Catheter ablation as first-line treatment for paroxysmal atrial fibrillation: A systematic review and meta-analysis. Heart. 2021;**107**(20):1630

[23] Hindricks G, Potpara T, Dagres N, Arbelo E, Bax JJ, Blomström-Lundqvist C, et al. 2020 ESC Guidelines for the diagnosis and management of atrial fibrillation developed in collaboration with the European Association for Cardio-Thoracic Surgery (EACTS): The Task Force for the diagnosis and management of atrial fibrillation of the European Society of Cardiology (ESC) Developed with the special contribution of the European Heart Rhythm Association (EHRA) of the ESC. European Heart Journal. 2021;**42**(5):373

[24] Kuck K-H, Brugada J, Fürnkranz A, Metzner A, Ouyang F, Chun G, et al. Cryoballoon or radiofrequency ablation for paroxysmal atrial fibrillation. New England Journal of Medicine. 2016;**374**:2235-2245

[25] Hachem AH, Marine JE, Tahboub HA, Kamdar S, Kanjwal S, Soni R, et al. Radiofrequency ablation versus cryoablation in the treatment of paroxysmal atrial fibrillation: A meta-analysis. Cardiology Research and Practice. 2018;**10**:6276241

[26] Khoueiry Z, Albenque J-P, Providencia R, Combes S, Combes N,

Jourda F, et al. Outcomes after cryoablation vs. radiofrequency in patients with paroxysmal atrial fibrillation: Impact of pulmonary veins anatomy. EP Europace. 2016;**18**:1343

[27] Kenneth Lauren Ripley, Andrew A. Gage, Don B. Olsen, John F. Vleet, Chu-Pak Lau, Hung-Fat TSE, Time Course of Esophageal Lesions After Catheter Ablation with Cryothermal and Radiofrequency Ablation Implication for Atrio-Esophageal Fistula Formation After Catheter Ablation for Atrial Fibrillation

[28] Gaynor SL, Ishii Y, Diodato MD, et al. Successful performance of Cox-maze procedure on beating heart using bipolar radiofrequency ablation: A feasibility study in animals. The Annals of Thoracic Surgery. 2004;**78**:1671-1677

[29] Lall SC, Melby SJ, Voeller RK, et al. The effect of ablation technology on surgical outcomes after the Cox-maze procedure: A propensity analysis. The Journal of Thoracic and Cardiovascular Surgery. 2007;**133**(2):389-396

[30] Weimar T, Schena S, Bailey MS, Maniar HS, Schuessler RB, Cox JL, et al. The Cox-maze procedure for lone atrial fibrillation: A single-center experience over 2 decades. Circulation. Arrhythmia and Electrophysiology. 2012;**5**:8-14

[31] Ad N, Holmes SD, Stone LE, Pritchard G, Henry L. Rhythm course over 5 years following surgical ablation for atrial fibrillation. European Journal of Cardio-Thoracic Surgery. Jan 2015;**47**(1):52-58; discussion 58. DOI: 10.1093/ejcts/ezu059. Epub 2014 Feb 28. PMID: 24585551

[32] Pet M, Robertson JO, Bailey M, Guthrie TJ, Moon MR, Lawton JS, et al. The impact of CHADS2 score on late stroke after the Cox maze procedure. The Journal of Thoracic and Cardiovascular Surgery. Jul 2013;**146**(1):85-89. DOI: 10.1016/j.jtcvs.2012.03.087. Epub 2012 Jul 19. PMID: 22818126; PMCID: PMC4369384

[33] Lawrance CP, Henn MC, Miller JR, Sinn LA, Schuessler RB, Damiano RJ Jr. Comparison of the stand-alone Cox-maze IV procedure to the concomitant Cox-maze IV and mitral valve procedure for atrial fibrillation. Ann Cardiothorac Surg. 2014;**3**:55-61

[34] Henn MC, Lawrance CP, Sinn LA, Miller JR, Schuessler RB, Moon MR, et al. Effectiveness of surgical ablation in patients with atrial fibrillation and aortic valve disease. The Annals of Thoracic Surgery. 2015;**100**:1253-1259

[35] Schill MR, Musharbash FN, Hansalia V, Greenberg JW, Melby SJ, Maniar HS, et al. Late results of the Cox-maze IV procedure in patients undergoing coronary artery bypass grafting. The Journal of Thoracic and Cardiovascular Surgery. 2017;**153**:1087-1094

[36] Lawrance CP, Henn MC, Miller JR, Sinn LA, Schuessler RB, Maniar HS, et al. A minimally invasive Cox maze IV procedure is as effective as sternotomy while decreasing major morbidity and hospital stay. The Journal of Thoracic and Cardiovascular Surgery. 2014;**148**:955-961

[37] Ruaengsri C, Schill MR, Khiabani AJ, Schuessler RB, Melby SJ, Damiano RJ. The Cox-maze IV procedure in its second decade: Still the gold standard? European Journal of Cardiothoracic Surgery. 2018;**53**:i19-i25

[38] Da Costa A et al. Robotic magnetic navigation for ablation of human arrhythmias. Medical Devices (Auckland, N.Z.). 2016;**9**:331-339

[39] Trippoli S, Di Spazio L, Chiumente M, Messori A. Medical therapy, radiofrequency ablation, or cryoballoon ablation as first-line treatment for paroxysmal atrial fibrillation: Interpreting efficacy through the shiny method. Cureus. 2022;**14**(2):e22645

[40] Aryana A, Morkoch S, Bailey S, Lim HW, Sara R, d'Avila A, et al. Acute procedural and cryoballoon characteristics from cryoablation of atrial fibrillation using the first- and second-generation cryoballoon: A retrospective comparative study with follow-up outcomes. Journal of Interventional Cardiac Electrophysiology. 2014;**41**(2):177-186

[41] Teunissen C, Velthuis BK, Hassink RJ, et al. Incidence of pulmonary vein stenosis after radiofrequency catheter ablation of atrial fibrillation. JACC Clinical Electrophysiology. Jun 2017;**3**(6):589-598. DOI: 10.1016/j.jacep.2017.02.003. Epub 2017 Apr 26. PMID: 29759432

Chapter 12

Left Atrial Appendage Closure for Stroke Prevention

Serkan Asil

Abstract

Atrial fibrillation is the most common chronic arrhythmia worldwide, and stroke is its most common complication. Approximately 20% of all ischemic strokes attributed to atrial fibrillation. Left atrial appendage thrombi are 90% responsible for embolic strokes in patients with non-valvular atrial fibrillation. In patients with atrial fibrillation, systemic anticoagulation is highly effective in lowering the risk of stroke. Bleeding problems and non-adherence hamper adequate anticoagulation therapy. As an alternative to stroke prevention with medical treatment, left atrial appendage closure is feasible and has proven to be an alternative to anticoagulation in non-valvular atrial fibrillation patients. Various left atrial appendage closure methods and devices have been defined and applied surgically and percutaneously. Exclusion of the left atrial appendage potentially minimizes the risk of embolic stroke and may eliminate chronic anticoagulation requirements. This chapter reviews left atrial appendage closure for stroke prevention in non-valvular atrial fibrillation.

Keywords: atrial fibrillation, left atrial appendage closure, stroke prevention

1. Introduction

Worldwide, atrial fibrillation (AF) is the most common sustained cardiac arrhythmia in adults [1]. The present prevalence of AF in adults is between 2% and 4%, with a 2.3-fold increase expected due to increased lifespan in the general population [1]. Increasing age is a main AF risk factor [2]. Additionally, the rising prevalence of other comorbidities and modifiable risk factors, such as hypertension (HT), diabetes mellitus (DM), heart failure (HF), coronary artery disease (CAD), chronic kidney disease (CKD), obesity, and obstructive sleep apnea (OSA), are critical [2]. Thromboembolic stroke in patients with atrial fibrillation may be attributed to the production and embolization of atrial thrombi, which primarily originate from the left atrial appendage.

Regardless of the treatment strategy of rate and rhythm control, treatment efforts must also focus on preventing thromboembolic events. The most vital complication attributed to AF is embolic stroke, and a meta-analysis of 50 studies detected AF in 24% of patients with embolic stroke of undetermined source [3]. Patients with AF are at high risk for thromboembolism, especially ischemic stroke. The risk of stroke in patients with non-valvular AF is approximately 5% per year [4]. Furthermore, compared to non-AF strokes, AF-related strokes are associated with increased mortality and morbidity, emphasizing the need of more effective stroke prevention in these patients.

The risk of stroke due to AF is specified by risk scores determined from population-based studies, and current guidelines recommend using the CHA_2DS_2VASc score for this purpose [2]. Based on the analysis of 1084 patients, Lip et al. validated this risk model and demonstrated incremental risk of embolic events with rising scores [5]. In patients with a risk score of 2 and above, oral anticoagulants (OAC) are recommended, considering the risk of bleeding. It can be recommended by evaluating the benefit-harm in patients with a score of 1 [2]. Many antithrombotic agents have been studied to prevent an ischemic stroke from AF. Studies that started with aspirin have shifted to

Anticoagulation strategy	Comparison group	Study name	Cerebral events risk	Comments
Aspirin	Placebo	Hart et al. (meta-analyses of six trials) [6].	Relative risk reduction 22% (CI 2–38)	Superiority of aspirin over placebo
Warfarin	Placebo	Hart et al. (meta-analyses of six trials) [6].	Relative risk reduction 62% (CI 48–72)	Superiority of warfarin over placebo
	Aspirin	Hart et al. (meta-analyses of five trials) [6].	Relative risk reduction 36% (CI 14–52)	Superiority of warfarin over aspirin
Dual Antiplatelet (Aspirin and clopidogrel)	Warfarin	Connolly et al. ACTIVE W [7].	Relative risk 1.44 (95% CI 1.18–1.76)	Trial stopped early due to benefit with warfarin
	Aspirin	Connolly et al. ACTIVE A [8].	Relative risk 0.72 (95% CI 0.62–0.83)	Bleeding risk 1.57 (95% CI 1.29–1.92)
Dabigatran 110 mg twice daily	Warfarin	Connolly et al. RELY [9].	Relative risk 0.91 (95% CI 0.74–1.11)	Bleeding risk is lower with dabigatran
Dabigatran 150 mg twice daily	Warfarin	Connolly et al. RELY [9].	Relative risk 0.66 (95% CI 0.53–0.82)	Bleeding risk is similar between groups
Rivaroxaban 20 mg daily	Warfarin	Patel et al. ROCKET AF [10].	Relative risk 0.79 (95% CI 0.66–0.96)	Similar overall bleeding, less intracranial/fatal
Apixaban 5 mg twice daily	Warfarin	Granger et al. ARISTOTLE [11].	Relative risk 0.79 (95% CI 0.66–0.95)	Less overall bleeding and all-cause mortality
Edoxaban 30 mg daily	Warfarin	Guigliano et al. ENGAGE-AF [12].	Relative risk 1.07 (95% CI 0.87–1.31)	Less bleeding and cardiovascular death
Edoxaban 60 mg daily	Warfarin	Guigliano et al. ENGAGE-AF [12].	Relative risk 0.79 (95% CI 0.63–0.99)	Less bleeding and cardiovascular death

Table 1.
Summary of antithrombotic therapy studies for stroke prevention in atrial fibrillation.

OAC agents with the clear benefit of warfarin in this area. Although long-term anticoagulation with warfarin is adequate, many drawbacks exist. The narrow therapeutic window complicates its use and compels a delicate balance between lack of efficacy and significantly elevated bleeding risk, and regular control blood tests are required. In addition, the presence of many drug and food interactions makes it more challenging to use in patients with advanced age and multisystem disease. In recent years, direct-acting anticoagulants (DOAC) (dabigatran, rivaroxaban, apixaban, edoxaban) that do not require routine monitoring have made a breakthrough in the treatment and have been used routinely. Antithrombotic therapy studies are briefly summarized in **Table 1**.

2. Left atrial appendage closure

In non-valvular atrial fibrillation, the thrombus originates in the left atrial appendage (LAA) in 90% of the patients [13]. The primary rationale for LAA closure is that the remaining small risk no longer warrants OAC after excluding the LAA as an embolic source. Exclusion of the LAA either by surgical or catheter-based means has been implemented in recent years.

LAA is the tubular blind-ended embryonic remnant of the left atrium, and its shape, number of lobes, depth, and orifice diameter varies and the risk of thrombus may vary according to these variables [14, 15]. Although it is known that LAA is an embryonic remnant, it also has some functions. For example, modulation of sympathetic and parasympathetic tone, decompression of the left atrium when atrial pressure rises, production of natriuretic peptide (primarily atrial natriuretic peptide), and contribution to the diastolic filling of the left ventricle [16].

Its complex shape with low-flow zones makes it prone to stasis, which can be seen in transesophageal echocardiography (TEE) as spontaneous echo contrast or reduced pulsed-wave velocity [17]. This change in the anatomy and hemodynamics of the LAA is of significant importance before the closure procedure. While direct visual evaluation may be acceptable in surgical closures, especially if percutaneous closure is planned, LAA diameter, depth, type, presence of thrombus, and interatrial septal anatomy should be evaluated in detail before the procedure with TEE, computed tomography (CT), and cardiac magnetic resonance imaging (MRI).

2.1 Surgical left atrial appendage closure

Surgical LAA exclusions were first performed in the 1940s but found limited application because they prolong the surgical procedure and require special techniques [18]. However, surgical techniques and devices have been developed in recent years, and LAA closure has been applied in patients who undergo cardiac surgery for other reasons if AF is accompanied. The only randomized controlled study on this subject, the Left Atrial Appendage Occlusion Study (LAAOS), was published in 2005 [19]. Seventy-seven patients with AF undergoing coronary artery bypass surgery were randomized 2:1 as LAA closure and LAA no closure. As a result of the study, it was specified that the procedure is safe, but the high rate of incomplete closure was not suitable for event evaluation [19]. In a retrospective study of 205 patients who underwent mitral valve replacement, a lower incidence of stroke was found in the group that underwent LAA closure (58 patients-52 had successful ligations) [20]. In light of this study data, the American College of Cardiology recommended considering LAA closure in AF patients who will undergo mitral valve surgery [21]. In a retrospective cohort study of 10,524 Medicare recipients with atrial fibrillation undergoing cardiac surgery, LAA closure resulted in a significant reduction in hospital admissions due to thromboembolism compared to non-closure (unadjusted, 4.2% vs. 6.2%; adjusted hazard ratio, 0.67) [22]. In a meta-analysis of five studies following had been analyzed – beneficial in one study, harmful in one study, and neutral in three studies, it was stated that there was not enough evidence for routine recommending closure. [23]. In this meta-analysis, incomplete closure rates were between 55 and 65%, and residual LAA flow or incomplete LAA closure may be associated with an increased risk of stroke [23, 24].

Surgical LAA closure or exclusion during cardiac surgery remains controversial for routine practice. The LAA structure is variable, and the risk of procedure complications increases due to its location close to the epicardial circumflex artery, the great cardiac vein, the endocardial mitral annulus, and the left upper pulmonary vein. European Society of Cardiology Atrial fibrillation guideline recommends that surgical occlusion or exclusion of the LAA be considered with class IIB recommendation level for stroke prevention in patients with AF undergoing cardiac surgery [2].

2.2 Catheter-based left atrial appendage closure

The primary downside to surgical LAA closure is that which holds little interest as a stand-alone procedure. The trials researching its utility included only patients undergoing cardiac surgery for another indication. Therefore, the appeal of a percutaneous procedure for closure of the LAA in patients at high risk for stroke and suboptimal candidates for anticoagulation because of hemorrhage is obvious and led to the development of the percutaneous catheter-based device systems. Percutaneous LAA closure has been applied since 2002 in Europe and since 2003 in the USA in patients with high thromboembolism risk and contraindications to OAC treatment.

There are two basic methods of LAA closure, endocardial and epicardial. LAA closure is performed by endovascular delivery of a nitinol-based device via a dedicated sheath inside the LAA. After the implant, antithrombotic treatment is required to prevent device-related thrombosis until endothelialization occurs. In percutaneous epicardial LAA exclusion, LAA closure is secondary to the epicardial ligation of the LAA. No foreign body is in touch with the bloodstream, and post-procedural antithrombotic treatment is usually undue unless a residual leak is present. Many devices have been developed for this purpose, the first of which is the Percutaneous LAA occluder (PLAATO, eV3, Inc., Plymouth, MA, USA) (**Figure 1**). The device was covered with a self-expanding nitinol cage and a non-thrombogenic PTFE membrane. Ostermayer et al. reported that PLAATO system implantation was performed on 111 non-valvular AF patients in a non-randomized, multi-center study [25]. The procedure was successfully terminated in 108 patients (97.3%). In a 6-month follow-up, a thrombus was detected on the device in one patient. In the successful long-term follow-up of 91 patients, stroke developed in two (2.2%) patients. In the 5-year results of the North American cohort of this study, the annual stroke rate of 64 patients was 3.8% in this population [26].

The WATCHMAN (Boston Scientific, Marlborough, MA, USA) is the other closure system most studied and has the only randomized controlled trial between LAA closure and warfarin (**Figure 1**). The WATCHMAN consists of a self-expanding Nitinol frame covered by a 160 μ m polyester membrane on its left atrial side. The device has a fixation barb around the mid-perimeter to secure the occlude to the left atrial

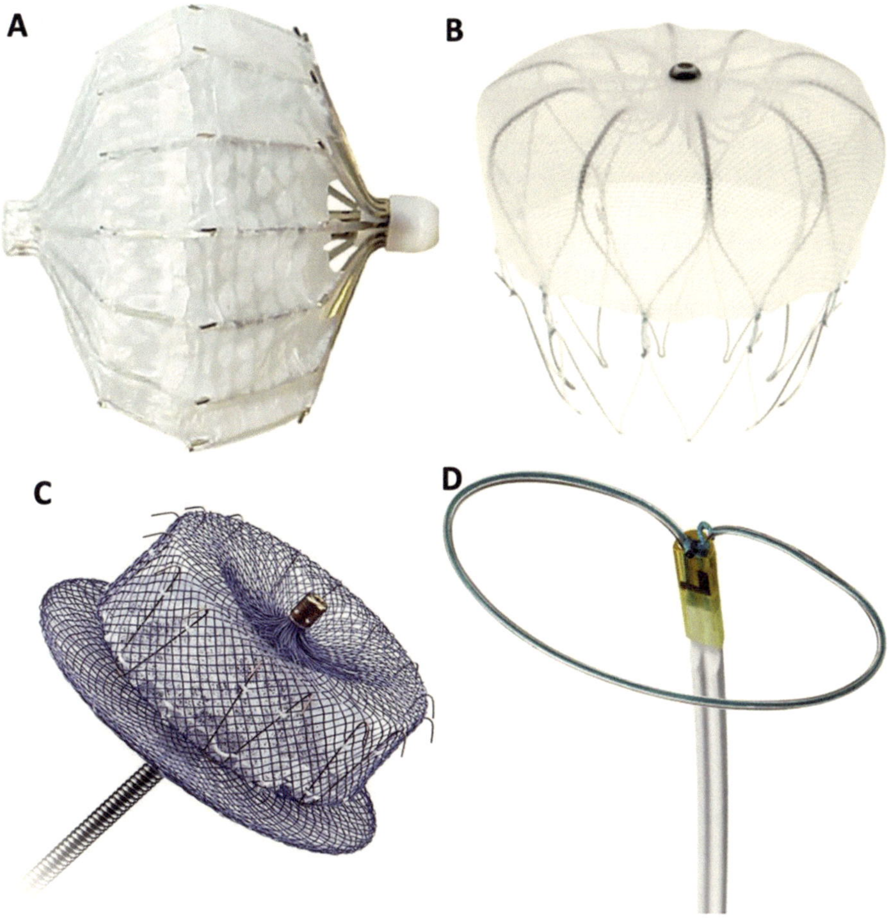

Figure 1.
A PLAATO device, B: WATCHMAN device, C: AMULET device, D; LARIAT device.

appendage wall. Measuring the width and length of the LAA before the procedure is essential to select the device diameter. There are five devices with diameters between 21 and 33 mm available to fit in different LAA ostium. The device's size should be 10–20% larger than the LAA ostium diameter.

The WATCHMAN LAA closure system was tested in a pilot study of 75 patients in terms of safety and efficacy, and the successful placement rate was found to be 88% [27]. Five of the first 16 patients developed device-related complications (two device embolization, one air embolism, one surgical device removal due to incorrect position, and one delivery system fracture requiring surgery) [27]. These complications led to design changes to the fixation barb and a second-generation device was used. No device embolization was found in other remaining 53 patients who have implemented a WATCHMAN device [27].

A prospective, randomized, multicenter PROTECT-AF study (percutaneous closure of the left atrial appendage versus warfarin therapy for prevention of stroke in patients with atrial fibrillation: a randomized non-inferiority trial) comparing LAA closure and long-term OAC therapy with the WATCHMAN LAA system with non-valvular AF (CHADS2 score ≥ 1), a total of 707 patients using OAC were randomized to the device and control groups in a 2:1 ratio [28]. This study had a non-inferiority design with a composite primary efficacy endpoint of cerebral events, cardiovascular death, and embolic event. In a mean follow-up of more than 1 year, the primary endpoint incidence was 3% in the device group, 4.9% in the OAC group, and the annual stroke rate was 2.3% in the device group and 3.2% in the OAC group [28]. Continued efficacy of the WATCHMAN device was demonstrated at a 4-year follow-up [29]. Procedural severe complications were observed in 12% of patients in the PROTECT-AF study. The most common severe complications are pericardial effusion (5%) requiring surgical or percutaneous intervention and acute stroke due to embolism (1.1%) [28].

Because of lingering safety concerns from the PROTECT AF trial, a second confirmatory trial, PREVAIL, randomized 407 patients 2:1 to device versus warfarin [30]. PREVAIL did not achieve non-inferiority for its primary efficacy outcome due to a low stroke rate in the control arm. At 18-months, the primary endpoint rate was 0.064 in the device group versus 0.063 in the control group (RR1.07, 0.95% CI 0.57–1.89) [30]. However, procedural complications decreased from 8.7% in PROTECT-AF to 4.2% in PREVAIL, especially rates of pericardial effusion requiring surgical repair decreased in this trial to 0.4% (compared to 1.6% in PROTECT AF) [30]. These findings led to the general conclusion that LAA closure is both safe and effective. A meta-analysis evaluating bleeding outcomes for the 1.114 patients enrolled in PROTECT AF and PREVAIL over the median of 3.1 years of follow-up showed similar overall bleeding rates between groups (3.5 vs. 3.6 events per 100 patient-years, RR 0.95, 95% CI 0.66–1.40 $p = 0.84$) [31]. However, there were significantly fewer ischemic events in LAA closure (1.8 vs. 3.6 events per 100 patient-years RR 0.49, 95%CI 0.32–0.75 $p = 0.001$) [31]. Furthermore, the combined 5-year PROTECT-AF and PREVAIL results demonstrated a numerically higher ischemic stroke, but this difference did not reach statistical significance (HR: 1.71; $p = 0.080$), also reductions in major bleeding, hemorrhagic stroke, and mortality in the device arm [32].

The EWOLUTION, a prospective, multicenter, single-arm registry, included 1020 patients undergoing WATCHMAN implantation that was designed to assess the real-world impact of LAA closure [33]. Thromboembolic and bleeding risk scores were higher in patients than in randomized controlled trials. After a median of 2 years of follow-up, the ischemic stroke rate was 83% lower than expected by the CHA_2DS_2VASc score. According to documented data, the major bleeding rate was reduced by 46% compared to normal rates when warfarin was used. The implant success was high (98.5%), and procedure and device-related adverse severe events ≤7 days were seen in 2.8% of patients (including death 0.4%; major bleeding 0.9%; tamponade 0.3%; device embolization 0.2%) [33].

The WATCHMAN FLX is a next-generation LAA closure device in the WATCHMAN family. In its US-approval trial (PINNACLE FLX), Watchman FLX has demonstrated equally favorable efficacy and safety profile [34].

LAA closure has also been performed using the Amplatzer devices. The Amplatzer Cardiac Plug (ACP) is a device developed specifically for LAA closure. In the first European experience with the ACP device, LAA closure was successfully performed in 132/137 patients (96%). Serious complications were seen in 10 (7%) patients in the first 24 hours [35]. In a multicenter retrospective study that investigated the safety, feasibility, and efficacy of the ACP device, 1047 patients were evaluated [36]. The success rate of the procedure was 97.3%. There were 52 (4.97%) periprocedural significant adverse events. In 1001/1019 (98.2%) of successfully implanted patients, follow-up was completed (average 13 months, total 1349 patient-years). All-cause mortality was 4.2% after one year. At the follow-up, no deaths were attributed to the device. During the follow-up period, there were nine strokes (0.9%) and nine transient ischemic attacks (0.9%) [36].

The Amplatzer AMULET (**Figure 1**) is an iterative design advance on the original ACP device. The configuration maintains the concept and the basic structure of the original version but was intended to improve device performance and increase the device's safety (including sealing and stability). The Amulet is a self-expanding nitinol device with two pre-mounted components (a lobe and a disc) on a single cable. The external disc provides more appropriate coverage of the LAA ostium. The distal lobe comprises of six to 10 pairs of stabilizing hooks across its diameter to anchor to the LAA and provide stability, which is enhanced by its gentle radial force and proximal disc traction. The most extensive study with the AMULET, LAA closure device, was an observational registry study [37]. In the study that included 1088 patients, AMULET was successfully implanted in 99% of cases. In TEE performed 1 to 3 months after the procedure, residual flow in the LAA was not observed in 98.4% of patients. The observed ischaemic stroke rate was 2.9% per year. Device-related thrombus was reported in 1.7% of patients [37].

AMULET IDE trial was designed to evaluate the safety and effectiveness of the Amulet LAA closure compared with the Watchman device [38]. The trial was designed for 1:1 randomized and multicenter, and 1878 patients enrolled in study. The AMULET device was non-inferior to the Watchman device for the primary safety endpoint (14.5% versus 14.7%; difference = −0.14 [95% CI, −3.42 to 3.13]; $P < 0.001$ for noninferiority). Major bleeding and all-cause death were similar among groups (10.6% versus 10.0% and 3.9% versus 5.1%, respectively). Procedure-related

Device	Design	Size	Proper LAA characteristics	Delivery System	Approval
Watchman (Endocardial) (Boston Scientific)	Single lobe	20–24–27-31-35	15 to 32 mm, width 1/2 device size, depth	14-Fr sheath; single-curve or double-curve	CE Mark (2005); FDA (2015)
Amulet (Endocardial) (Abbott)	Distal lobe and proximal disc	16, 18, 20, 22, 25, 28, 31, and 34	11 to 31 mm, width > 12 to 15 mm, depth	12-Fr or 14-Fr sheath; double curve	CE Mark (2013)
LAmbre (Lifetech Scientific Co., Ltd.)	Double (umbrella and cover)	16, 18, 20, 22, 24, 26, 28, 30, 32, 34, 36	The size of the implant would be 4 to 8 mm larger than the measured LAA orifice.	8–10- Fr sheath	CE Mark (2016);
Ultraseal (Cardia Inc.)	Double (bulb and sail)	16, 18, 20, 22, 24, 26, 28, 30, 32	Maximum measured landing zone, with ≥25% oversizing.	10–12-Fr sheath	CE Mark (2016)
Lariat (Epicardial) (SentreHeart)	Non-absorbable suture	40 and 45 (suture loop)	Up to 40 mm width Up to 70 mm length.	13.5-Fr epicardial sheath; 8.5-Fr endocardial sheath; magnet-tip wires; endocardial balloon	CE Mark (2015); FDA 510(k) (2006), surgical use only

Table 2.
Most common left atrial appendage closure devices and main characteristics.

Device	Trial	Study design	Number	Implant success	Procedure-related complications	Systemic thromboembolism
Watchman (Endocardial) (Boston Scientific)	PROTECT AF 2009 [28]	Randomized control trial	707 patients 2:1 randomization	91%	12%	3 events per 100 patient years.
	PREVAIL 2014 [30]	Randomized control trial	407 patients 2:1 randomization	95%	5%	2%
	EWOLUTION 2017 [33]	Prospective observational	1020	99%	3%	2%
	Reddy et al. 2017 [32]	Prospective observational	3822	96%	2%	—
Amulet (Endocardial) (Abbott)	Landmesser et al. 2017 [37]	Prospective observational	1088	99%	6%	3% per year
LAmbre (Lifetech Scientific Co., Ltd.)	Huang et al. 2017 [39]	Prospective observational	153	99%	6%	1%
Lariat (Epicardial) (SentreHeart)	Lakkireddy et al. 2016 [40]	Retrospective observational	712	94%	!0%	—

Table 3.
Main studies of percutaneous left atrial appendage closure devices.

complications were higher for the AMULET device (4.5% versus 2.5%), primarily related to more frequent pericardial effusion and device embolization [38].

Other less common endocardial LAA closure devices are WAVECREST (Biosense Webster, Diamond Bar, CA, USA), LAMBRE (Lifetech Scientific, Shenzhen, China), ULTRASEAL (Cardia Inc. – Eagan, MN, USA), OCCLUTECH (Occlutech International. **Tables 2** and **3** summarize left atrial appendix closure device features and main study results.

LARİAT (SentreHeart, Redwood City, CA, USA) is a suture-based LAA exclusion device that allows epicardial LAA ligation with no device left in the endocardial area. Therefore, LAA occlusion is secondary to the epicardial ligation of the LAA. In the multicenter observational registry study concerning 712 patients, LARIAT was successfully performed in 682 patients (95.5%) [40]. The complete exclusion was achieved in 669 patients (98%), while 13 patients (1.8%) had a trace leak (<2 mm). There was one death related to the procedure. Ten patients (1.44%) had cardiac perforation necessitating open surgery, while another 14 (2.01%) did not require surgery. Delayed complications (pericarditis, pericardial and pleural effusion) occurred in 34 (4.78%) [40].

In clinical practice, the most prevalent reason for LAA occlusion/exclusion is a perceived high bleeding risk or less frequently contraindications to OAC. On the other hand, LAA closure devices have not been tested in such groups at random. Most patients who would have been considered inappropriate for OAC treatment with warfarin a few years ago now seem to do well on DOAC, and LAA closure has not been compared to DOAC therapy or surgical LAA occlusion/exclusion in patients at risk for bleeding. In patients with anticoagulation contraindications, appropriately powered trials are needed to determine the optimum LAA closure indications compared to DOAC therapy [2]. The 2020 European Society of Cardiology Atrial Fibrillation guidelines recommends catheter-based LAA closure with class IIB level [2].

3. Procedure

Pre-procedural imaging is required to rule out LAA thrombus, examine LAA anatomy for appropriateness for percutaneous closure, and identify the optimal device sizing. Left atrial appendage thrombus is not an absolute contraindication for LAA closure. It has been reported that closure is performed by experienced operators, especially in the presence of a deeply located organized thrombus [41, 42]. The LAA is viewed in many planes with TEE, the most common being 0°, 45°, 90°, and 135° angles [43]. As a result, the maximum LAA dimensions for the LAA closure device are estimated (**Figure 2**). In addition, CT can be used. It offers a higher spatial resolution than TEE, allowing the 3D reconstruction of vital anatomical structures, and LAA thrombi can be ruled out safely with delayed acquisition imaging [44] (**Figure 3**). Each LAA closing device has different measurement areas and details to match its specifications. Since the AMULET device is used in our center, we used images of LAA sizing for AMULET in TEE, and procedural images of the device implantation.

The procedure should be performed under general anesthesia, and patients could be intubated for optimal TEE guidance. Fluoroscopy and three-dimensional (3D) TEE assistance should be used to accomplish transseptal puncture. If no anatomic changes hindered optimal alignment, the transseptal puncture should be performed at the inferoposterior site of the interatrial septum. Also, it is possible to utilize intracardiac echocardiography (ICE) during the implant procedure [45]. After a successful

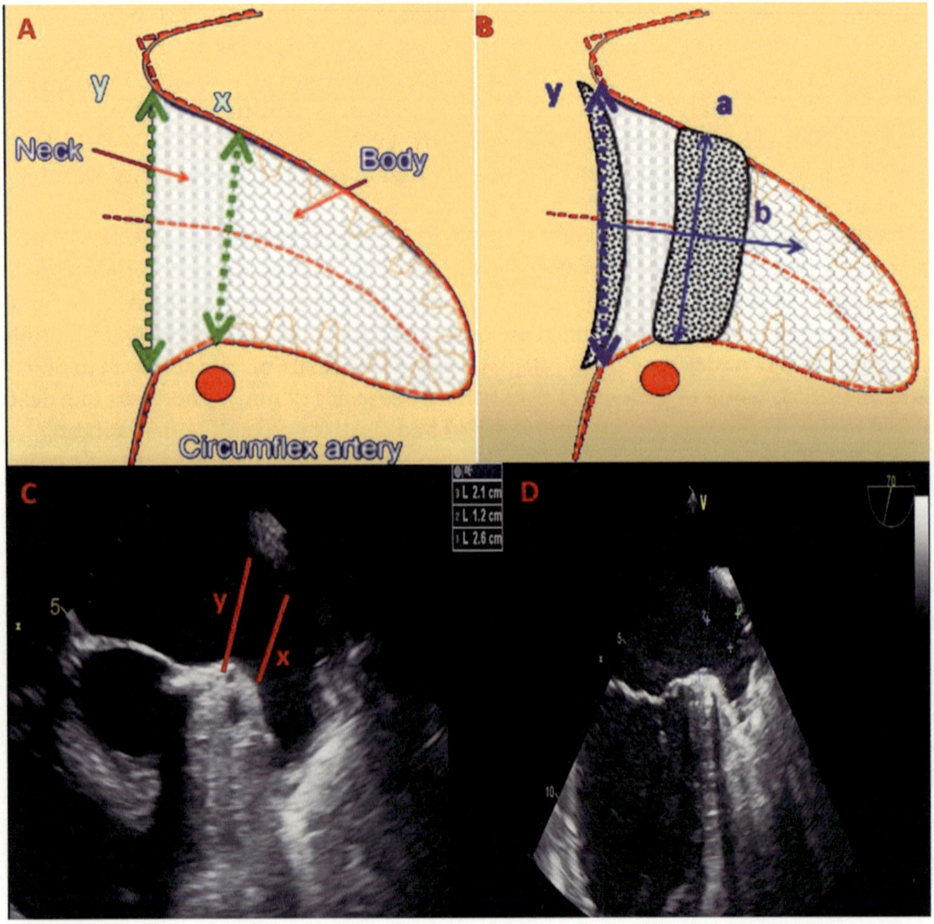

Figure 2.
Preprocedural left atrial appendage sizing with transesophageal echocardiography (for AMULET device).

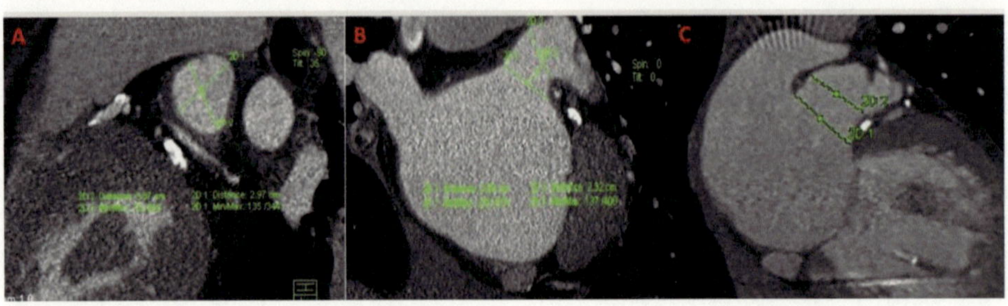

Figure 3.
Preprocedural left atrial appendage anatomy and diameter evaluation and device sizing with cardiac computed tomography (for AMULET device).

transseptal puncture, the delivery catheter can be inserted in the left atrium. Once the delivery catheter is engaged in LAA, LAA angiography is performed to confirm its size, usually using an RAO caudal projection, which is roughly equivalent to a 135°

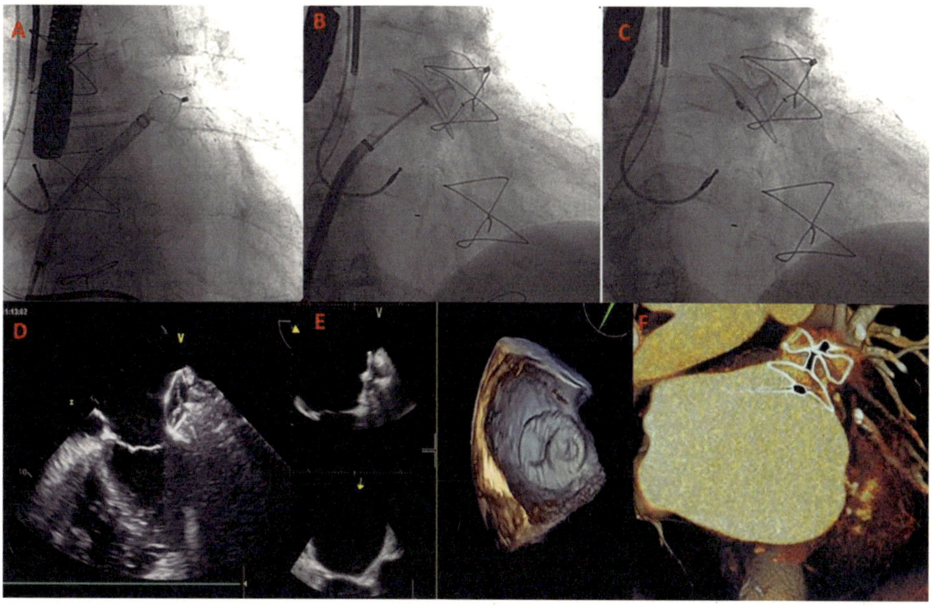

Figure 4.
A-E; LAA closure procedure with the fluoroscopy and transesophageal echocardiographic guidance. F: Postprocedural device image in cardiac computed tomography.

TEE view. For optimal sizing and safe sheath positioning, different views may be required. The deployment of LAA closure devices is done slowly and cautiously. After the device is positioned in the LAA, it is placed by unsheathing. LAA closure devices should be evaluated for proper alignment, compression, the absence of any peri-device leak, and stability before being released (the "tug test") (**Figure 4**).

The patient must be treated with a combination of anti-thrombotic drugs (anti-platelet and/or anticoagulation) following the procedure, with the specific regimen being determined by the LAA closure device utilized and matched to the patient's individual bleeding risk [46]. Complications related to LAAO are primarily acute; most of them can be detected by peri-procedural imaging. Cardiac perforation, pericardial effusion/tamponade, procedure-related stroke, and device embolization are common acute complications. In the late period of device implantation, device-related thrombosis and residual leakage-associated stroke can be seen. Surveillance imaging is needed to ensure proper LAA closure and the absence of device-related thrombosis at follow-up. TEE is the preferred imaging method because it gives real-time flow information without exposing the patient to radiation.

4. Conclusion

As a result, LAA closure is a proven treatment method with safety and effectiveness against warfarin. However, only the Watchman device has randomized controlled trials, other devices do not have randomized controlled trials yet, and current evidence was acquired from the registry and observational data. Furthermore, anticoagulants used in AF patients are mostly DOACs, and there is no randomized controlled study comparing DOACs. Despite these shortcomings, percutaneous LAA closure may be a good alternative for patients who are not suitable for anticoagulation or experience life-threatening bleeding with anticoagulants.

Acknowledgements

I want to thank Hacettepe University Cardiology Clinic for letting me use their case images.

Conflict of interest

The authors declare no conflict of interest.

Author details

Serkan Asil
Gülhane Training and Research Hospital Department of Cardiology, Ankara, Turkey

*Address all correspondence to: dr_serkanasil@hotmail.com

References

[1] Tsao CW, Aday AW, Almarzooq ZI, Alonso A, Beaton AZ, Bittencourt MS, et al. Heart disease and stroke statistics—2022 update: A report from the American Heart Association. Circulation. 2022;**145**:e153-e639

[2] Hindricks G, Potpara T, Dagres N, Arbelo E, Bax JJ, Blomström-Lundqvist C, et al. 2020 ESC guidelines for the diagnosis and management of atrial fibrillation developed in collaboration with the European Association for Cardio-Thoracic Surgery (EACTS): The task force for the diagnosis and management of atrial fibrillation of the European Society of Cardiology (ESC) developed with the special contribution of the European heart rhythm association (EHRA) of the ESC. European Heart Journal. 2020;**42**:373-498

[3] Sposato LA, Cipriano LE, Saposnik G, Vargas ER, Riccio PM, Hachinski V. Diagnosis of atrial fibrillation after stroke and transient ischaemic attack: A systematic review and meta-analysis. The Lancet Neurology. 2015;**14**:377-387

[4] Laupacis A, Boysen G, Connolly S, Ezekowitz M, Hart R, James K, et al. Risk factors for stroke and efficacy of antithrombotic therapy in atrial fibrillation. Analysis of pooled data from five randomized controlled trials. Archives of Internal Medicine. 1994;**154**:1449-1457

[5] Lip GY, Nieuwlaat R, Pisters R, Lane DA, Crijns HJ. Refining clinical risk stratification for predicting stroke and thromboembolism in atrial fibrillation using a novel risk factor-based approach: The euro heart survey on atrial fibrillation. Chest. 2010;**137**:263-272

[6] Hart RG, Benavente O, McBride R, Pearce LA. Antithrombotic therapy to prevent stroke in patients with atrial fibrillation: A meta-analysis. Annals of Internal Medicine. 1999;**131**:492-501

[7] Site HG. Clopidogrel plus aspirin versus oral anticoagulation for atrial fibrillation in the atrial fibrillation Clopidogrel trial with Irbesartan for prevention of vascular events (ACTIVE W): A randomised controlled trial. Lancet. 2006;**367**:1903-1912

[8] Investigators A. Effect of clopidogrel added to aspirin in patients with atrial fibrillation. New England Journal of Medicine. 2009;**360**:2066-2078

[9] Connolly SJ, Ezekowitz MD, Yusuf S, Eikelboom J, Oldgren J, Parekh A, et al. Dabigatran versus warfarin in patients with atrial fibrillation. The New England Journal of Medicine. 2009;**361**:1139-1151

[10] Patel MR, Mahaffey KW, Garg J, Pan G, Singer DE, Hacke W, et al. Rivaroxaban versus warfarin in nonvalvular atrial fibrillation. The New England Journal of Medicine. 2011;**365**:883-891

[11] Granger CB, Alexander JH, McMurray JJ, Lopes RD, Hylek EM, Hanna M, et al. Apixaban versus warfarin in patients with atrial fibrillation. The New England Journal of Medicine. 2011;**365**:981-992

[12] Giugliano RP, Ruff CT, Braunwald E, Murphy SA, Wiviott SD, Halperin JL, et al. Edoxaban versus warfarin in patients with atrial fibrillation. The New England Journal of Medicine. 2013;**369**:2093-2104

[13] Blackshear JL, Odell JA. Appendage obliteration to reduce stroke in cardiac

surgical patients with atrial fibrillation. The Annals of Thoracic Surgery. 1996;**61**:755-759

[14] Veinot JP, Harrity PJ, Gentile F, Khandheria BK, Bailey KR, Eickholt JT, et al. Anatomy of the normal left atrial appendage: A quantitative study of age-related changes in 500 autopsy hearts: Implications for echocardiographic examination. Circulation. 1997;**96**:3112-3115

[15] Di Biase L, Santangeli P, Anselmino M, Mohanty P, Salvetti I, Gili S, et al. Does the left atrial appendage morphology correlate with the risk of stroke in patients with atrial fibrillation? Results from a multicenter study. Journal of the American College of Cardiology. 2012;**60**:531-538

[16] Al-Saady N, Obel O, Camm A. Left atrial appendage: Structure, function, and role in thromboembolism. Heart. 1999;**82**:547-554

[17] Tamura H, Watanabe T, Nishiyama S, Sasaki S, Wanezaki M, Arimoto T, et al. Prognostic value of low left atrial appendage wall velocity in patients with ischemic stroke and atrial fibrillation. Journal of the American Society of Echocardiography. 2012;**25**:576-583

[18] Madden JL. Resection of the left auricular appendix: A prophylaxis for recurrent arterial emboli. Journal of the American Medical Association. 1949;**140**:769-772

[19] Healey JS, Crystal E, Lamy A, Teoh K, Semelhago L, Hohnloser SH, et al. Left atrial appendage occlusion study (LAAOS): Results of a randomized controlled pilot study of left atrial appendage occlusion during coronary bypass surgery in patients at risk for stroke. American Heart Journal. 2005;**150**:288-293

[20] Mn G-F. Pérez-David E, Quiles J, Peralta J, García-Rojas I, Bermejo J, Moreno M, Silva J: Role of left atrial appendageobliteration in stroke reductionin patients with mitral valve prosthesis: A transesophageal echocardiographic study. Journal of the American College of Cardiology. 2003;**42**:1253-1258

[21] January CT, Wann LS, Alpert JS, Calkins H, Cigarroa JE, Cleveland JC, et al. 2014 AHA/ACC/HRS guideline for the Management of Patients with Atrial Fibrillation. Circulation. 2014;**130**:e199-e267

[22] Friedman DJ, Piccini JP, Wang T, Zheng J, Malaisrie SC, Holmes DR, et al. Association between left atrial appendage occlusion and readmission for thromboembolism among patients with atrial fibrillation undergoing concomitant cardiac surgery. JAMA. 2018;**319**:365-374

[23] Dawson AG, Asopa S, Dunning J. Should patients undergoing cardiac surgery with atrial fibrillation have left atrial appendage exclusion? Interactive Cardiovascular and Thoracic Surgery. 2010;**10**:306-311

[24] Aryana A, Singh SK, Singh SM, O'Neill PG, Bowers MR, Allen SL, et al. Association between incomplete surgical ligation of left atrial appendage and stroke and systemic embolization. Heart Rhythm. 2015;**12**:1431-1437

[25] Ostermayer SH, Reisman M, Kramer PH, Matthews RV, Gray WA, Block PC, et al. Percutaneous left atrial appendage transcatheter occlusion (PLAATO system) to prevent stroke in high-risk patients with non-rheumatic atrial fibrillation: Results from the international multi-center feasibility trials. Journal of the American College of Cardiology. 2005;**46**:9-14

[26] Block PC, Burstein S, Casale PN, Kramer PH, Teirstein P, Williams DO, et al. Percutaneous left atrial appendage occlusion for patients in atrial fibrillation suboptimal for warfarin therapy: 5-year results of the PLAATO (percutaneous left atrial appendage Transcatheter occlusion) study. JACC. Cardiovascular Interventions. 2009;**2**:594-600

[27] Sick PB, Schuler G, Hauptmann KE, Grube E, Yakubov S, Turi ZG, et al. Initial worldwide experience with the WATCHMAN left atrial appendage system for stroke prevention in atrial fibrillation. Journal of the American College of Cardiology. 2007;**49**:1490-1495

[28] Holmes DR, Reddy VY, Turi ZG, Doshi SK, Sievert H, Buchbinder M, et al. Percutaneous closure of the left atrial appendage versus warfarin therapy for prevention of stroke in patients with atrial fibrillation: A randomised non-inferiority trial. Lancet. 2009;**374**:534-542

[29] Reddy VY, Sievert H, Halperin J, Doshi SK, Buchbinder M, Neuzil P, et al. Percutaneous left atrial appendage closure vs warfarin for atrial fibrillation: A randomized clinical trial. JAMA. 2014;**312**:1988-1998

[30] Holmes DR Jr, Kar S, Price MJ, Whisenant B, Sievert H, Doshi SK, et al. Prospective randomized evaluation of the Watchman left atrial appendage closure device in patients with atrial fibrillation versus long-term warfarin therapy: The PREVAIL trial. Journal of the American College of Cardiology. 2014;**64**:1-12

[31] Price MJ, Reddy VY, Valderrábano M, Halperin JL, Gibson DN, Gordon N, et al. Bleeding outcomes after left atrial appendage closure compared with long-term warfarin: A pooled, patient-level analysis of the WATCHMAN randomized trial experience. JACC. Cardiovascular Interventions. 2015;**8**:1925-1932

[32] Reddy VY, Doshi SK, Kar S, Gibson DN, Price MJ, Huber K, et al. 5-year outcomes after left atrial appendage closure: From the PREVAIL and PROTECT AF trials. Journal of the American College of Cardiology. 2017;**70**:2964-2975

[33] Boersma LV, Ince H, Kische S, Pokushalov E, Schmitz T, Schmidt B, et al. Evaluating real-world clinical outcomes in atrial fibrillation patients receiving the WATCHMAN left atrial appendage closure technology: Final 2-year outcome data of the EWOLUTION trial focusing on history of stroke and hemorrhage. Circulation. Arrhythmia and Electrophysiology. 2019;**12**:e006841

[34] Kar S, Doshi SK, Sadhu A, Horton R, Osorio J, Ellis C, et al. Primary outcome evaluation of a next-generation left atrial appendage closure device: Results from the PINNACLE FLX trial. Circulation. 2021;**143**:1754-1762

[35] Park JW, Bethencourt A, Sievert H, Santoro G, Meier B, Walsh K, et al. Left atrial appendage closure with Amplatzer cardiac plug in atrial fibrillation: Initial European experience. Catheterization and Cardiovascular Interventions. 2011;**77**:700-706

[36] Tzikas A, Shakir S, Gafoor S, Omran H, Berti S, Santoro G, et al. Left atrial appendage occlusion for stroke prevention in atrial fibrillation: Multicentre experience with the AMPLATZER cardiac plug. EuroIntervention. 2016;**11**:1170-1179

[37] Landmesser U, Tondo C, Camm J, Diener HC, Paul V, Schmidt B, et al. Left atrial appendage occlusion with

the AMPLATZER amulet device: One-year follow-up from the prospective global amulet observational registry. EuroIntervention. 2018;**14**:e590-e597

[38] Lakkireddy D, Thaler D, Ellis CR, Swarup V, Sondergaard L, Carroll J, et al. Amplatzer amulet left atrial appendage Occluder versus Watchman device for stroke prophylaxis (amulet IDE): A randomized, Controlled Trial. Circulation. 2021;**144**:1543-1552

[39] Huang H, Liu Y, Xu Y, Wang Z, Li Y, Cao K, et al. Percutaneous left atrial appendage closure with the LAmbre device for stroke prevention in atrial fibrillation: A prospective, Multicenter Clinical Study. JACC: Cardiovascular Interventions. 2017;**10**:2188-2194

[40] Lakkireddy D, Afzal MR, Lee RJ, Nagaraj H, Tschopp D, Gidney B, et al. Short and long-term outcomes of percutaneous left atrial appendage suture ligation: Results from a US multicenter evaluation. Heart Rhythm. 2016;**13**:1030-1036

[41] Aytemir K, Aminian A, Asil S, Canpolat U, Kaya EB, Şahiner L, et al. First case of percutaneous left atrial appendage closure by amulet™ device in a patient with left atrial appendage thrombus. International Journal of Cardiology. 2016;**223**:28-30

[42] Sahiner L, Coteli C, Kaya EB, Ates A, Kilic GS, Yorgun H, et al. Left atrial appendage occlusion in patients with thrombus in left atrial appendage. The Journal of Invasive Cardiology. 2020;**32**:222-227

[43] Altszuler D, Vainrib AF, Bamira DG, Benenstein RJ, Aizer A, Chinitz LA, et al. Left atrial occlusion device implantation: The role of the Echocardiographer. Current Cardiology Reports. 2019;**21**:66

[44] Korsholm K, Berti S, Iriart X, Saw J, Wang DD, Cochet H, et al. Expert recommendations on cardiac computed tomography for planning Transcatheter left atrial appendage occlusion. JACC. Cardiovascular Interventions. 2020;**13**:277-292

[45] Korsholm K, Jensen JM, Nielsen-Kudsk JE. Intracardiac echocardiography from the left atrium for procedural guidance of Transcatheter left atrial appendage occlusion. JACC. Cardiovascular Interventions. 2017;**10**:2198-2206

[46] Glikson M, Wolff R, Hindricks G, Mandrola J, Camm AJ, Lip GYH, et al. EHRA/EAPCI expert consensus statement on catheter-based left atrial appendage occlusion - an update. EuroIntervention. 2020;**15**:1133-1180